Intermittent Fasting *For* Women Over 40

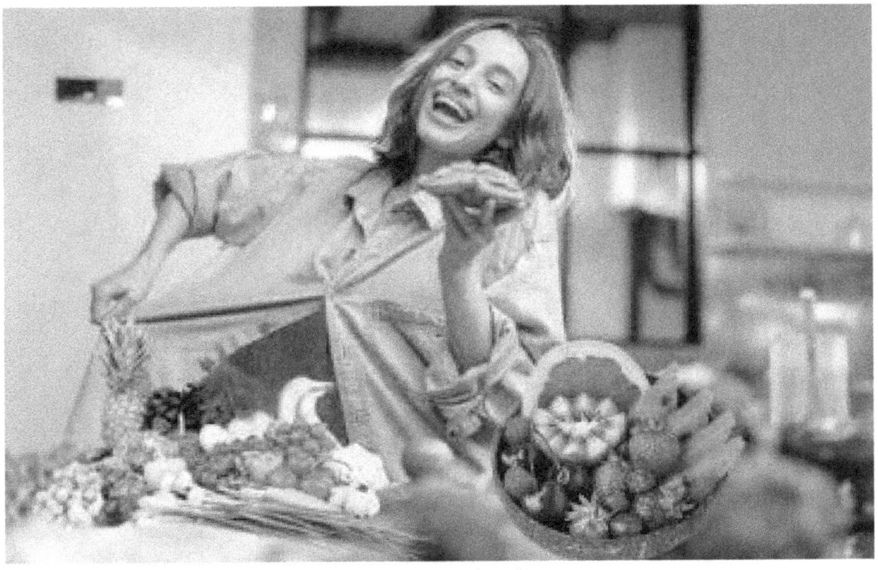

A Woman's Complete Guide to Using the Healing Power of Fasting to Burn Fat Boost Energy and Balance Immune System.

By

Jessica C. James

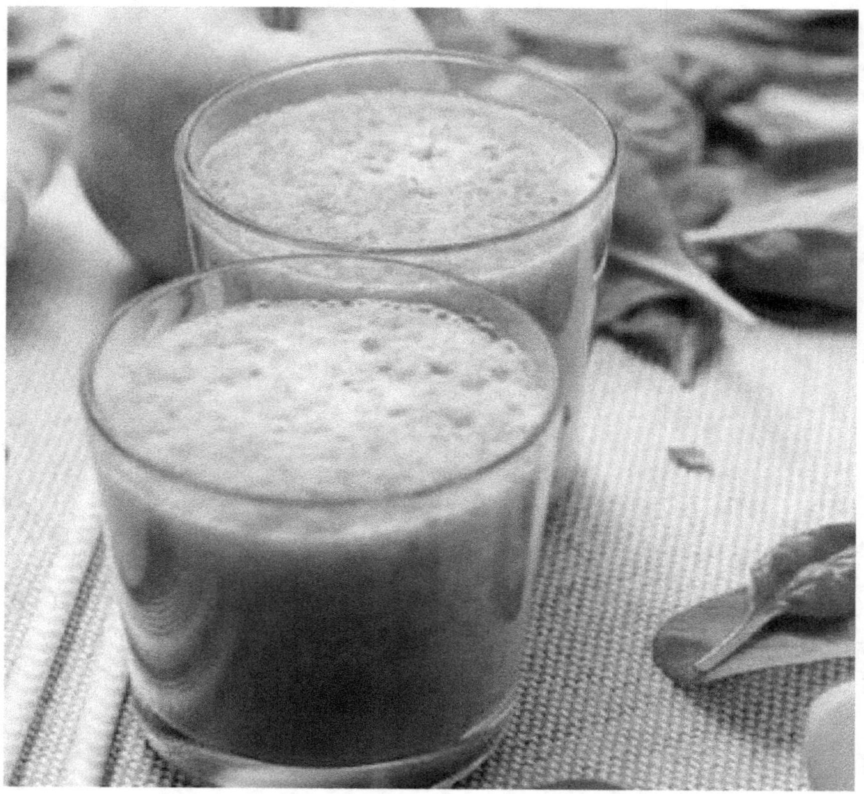

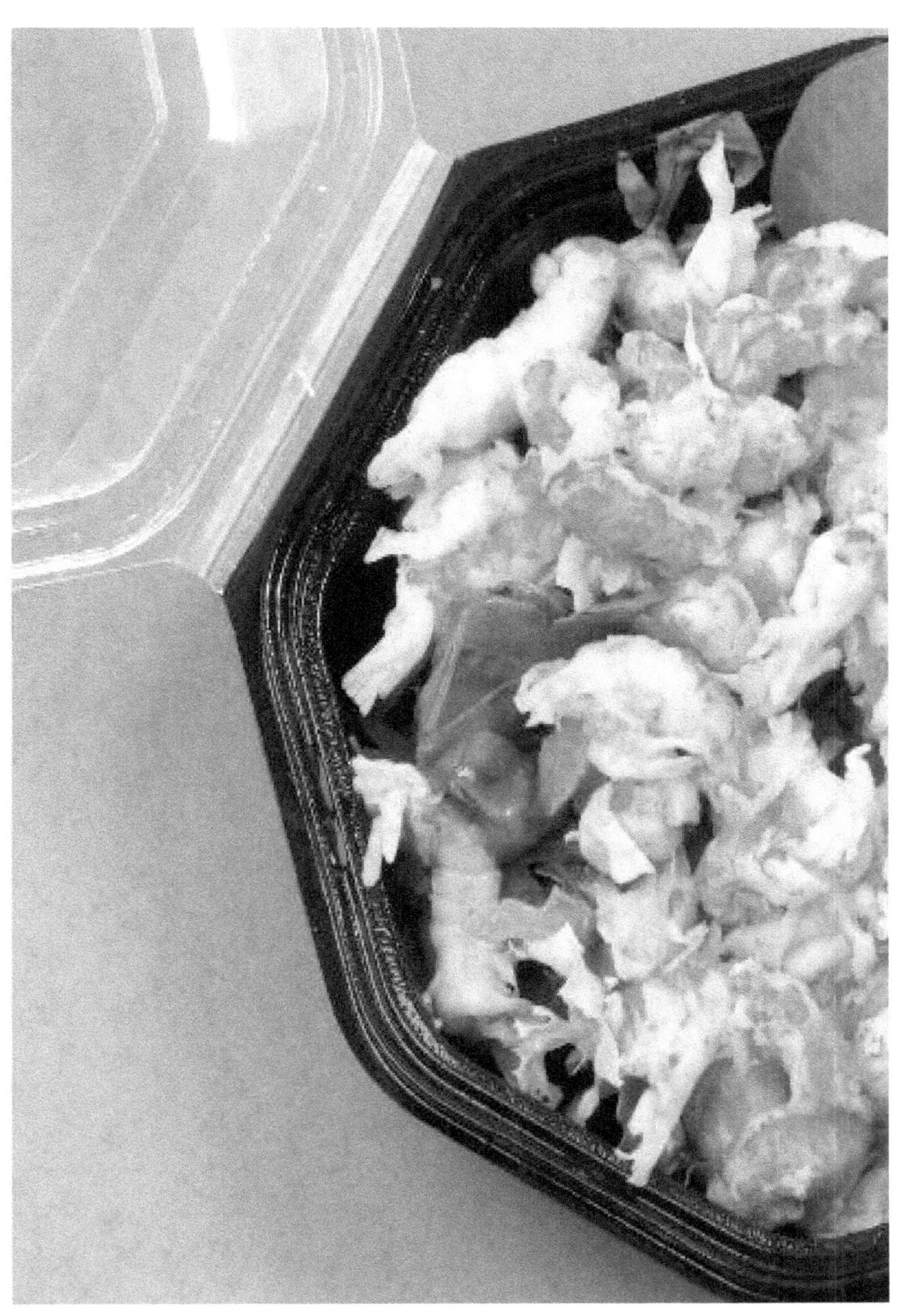

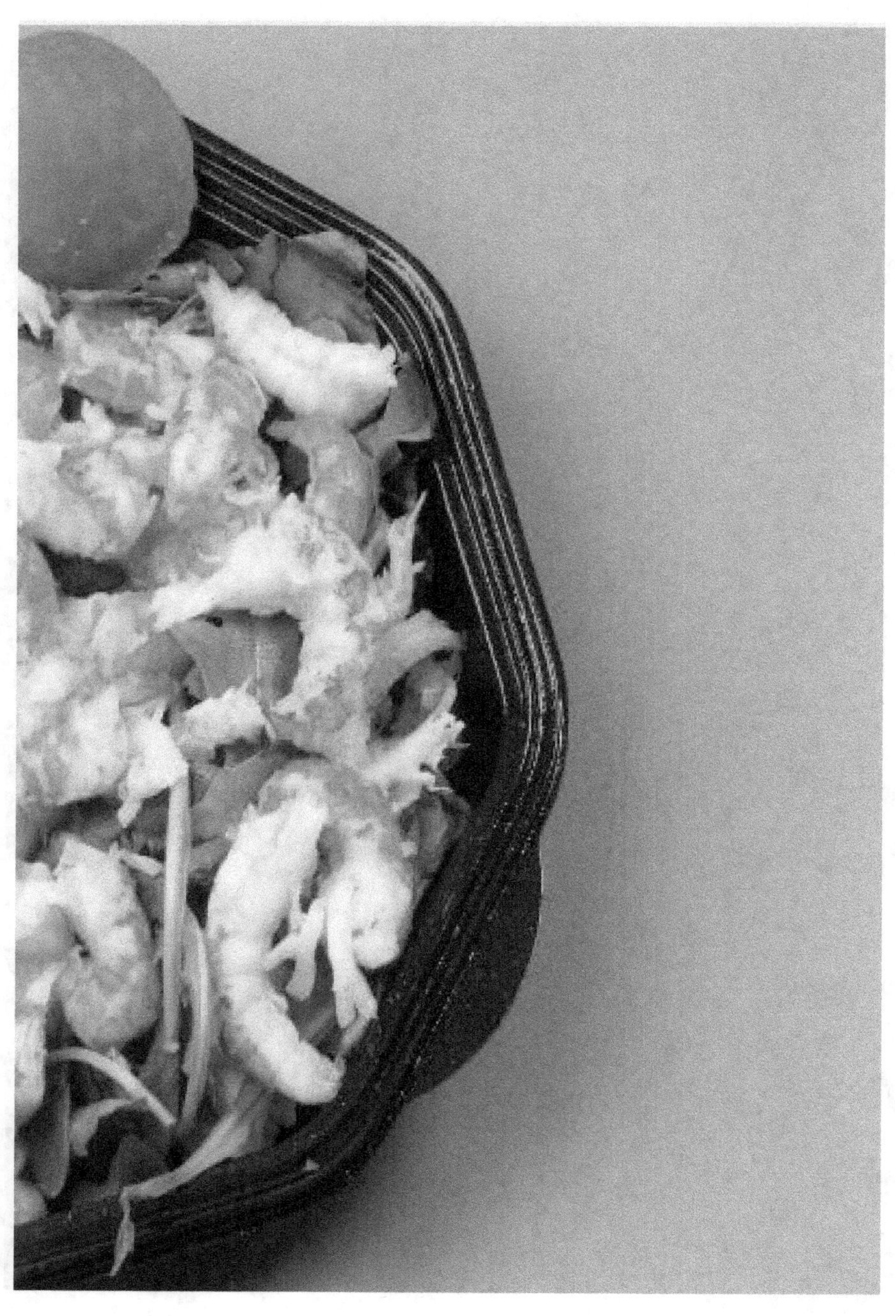

TABLE CONTENTS

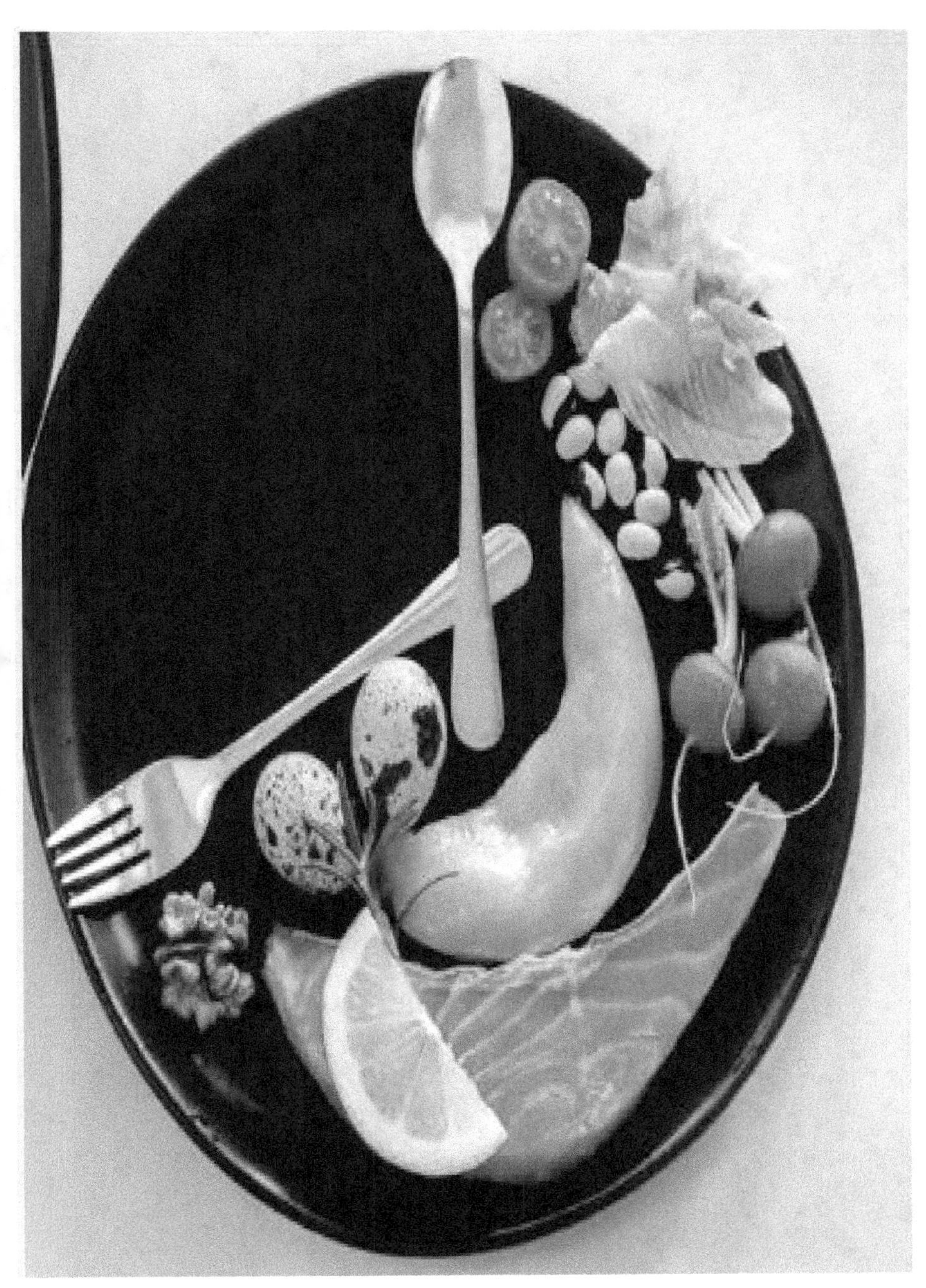

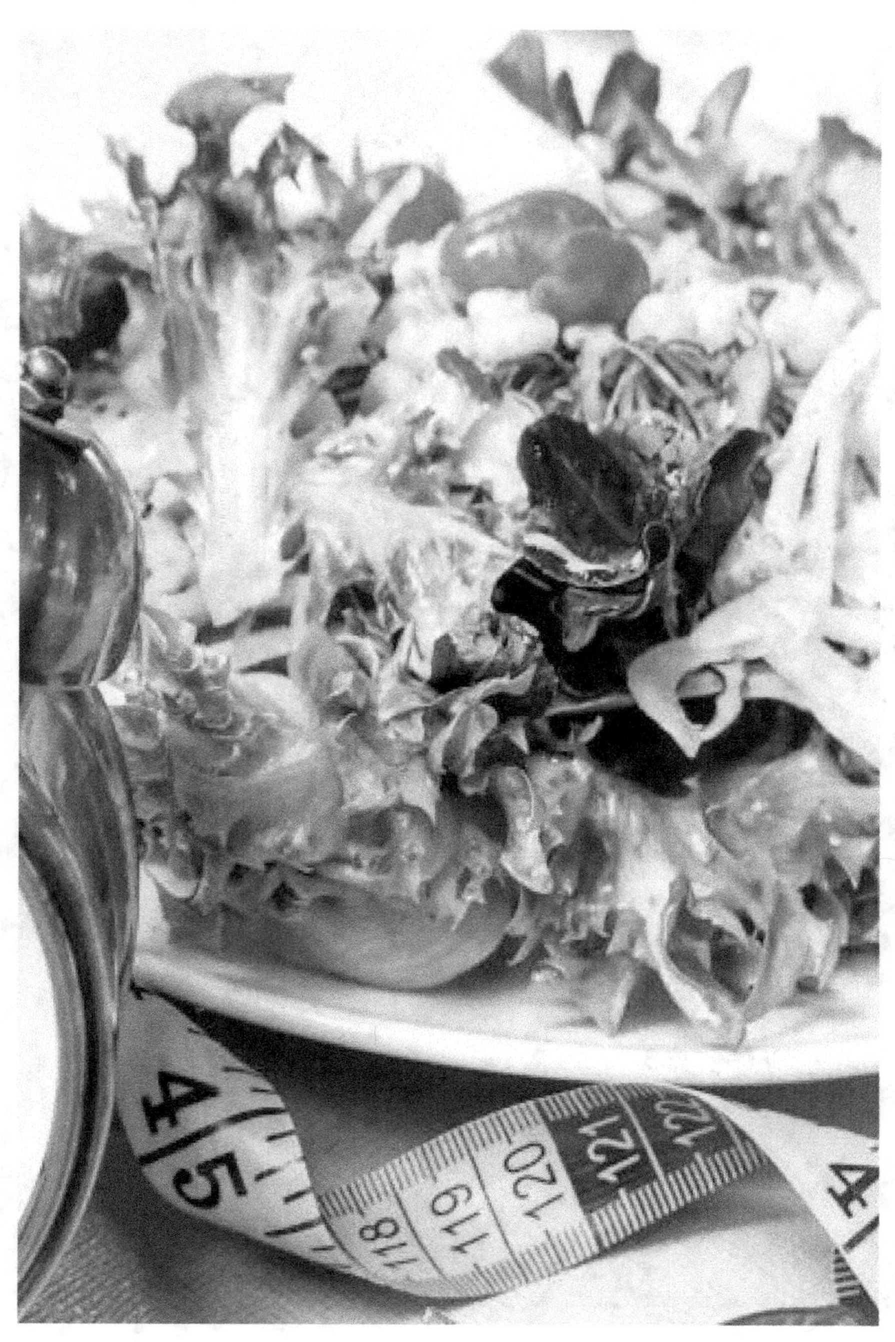

INTRODUCTION

Welcome to a journey that promises to transform not just your body, but your entire approach to health and well-being. This isn't just another diet book; it's a gateway to a lifestyle that thousands of women over 40, just like you, have found not only sustainable but life-changing.

Why intermittent fasting, and why now? The answer lies in understanding our bodies as they mature, recognizing that what worked in our twenties and thirties may not serve us as well in our forties and beyond.

As women, our bodies undergo profound changes as we age, from shifts in metabolism to the fluctuating tides of our hormones. It's time for a strategy that acknowledges and embraces these changes, rather than fighting against them.

Intermittent fasting offers a flexible, adaptable approach to health and wellness, one that can be tailored to fit your life, your goals, and your unique physiological needs at this stage. It's not about deprivation; it's about empowerment.

It's about learning to listen to your body, understanding its signals, and feeding it in a way that fuels not just physical health, but mental and emotional well-being.

This book is designed to be your companion on a journey of discovery. Together, we'll explore how intermittent fasting can help balance hormones, aid in weight management, enhance mental clarity, and contribute to longer, healthier living. We'll debunk myths, tackle common challenges, and provide you with the knowledge and tools you need to integrate fasting into your life in a way that feels natural and enjoyable.

But this book is about more than just fasting. It's about crafting a lifestyle that supports your goals. From nutrition and exercise to mindfulness and self-care, we'll cover all the bases, ensuring you have a comprehensive plan that works for you.

To the women over 40 who are reading this: know that it's never too late to make a change. Whether you're looking to improve your health, boost your energy levels, or simply feel better in your skin, this book is for you. Your journey to a healthier, happier you start right here, right now. Let's embark on this journey together.

ADDRESSING COMMON CONCERNS

When you're trying to make changes in your life, like starting a new diet or exercise plan, it's normal to have some worries or questions. Let's talk about some common concerns people have and offer simple ways to think about and handle them:

1. "Will I feel too hungry if I start fasting?"

It's normal to feel a bit hungrier when you first start fasting because your body is getting used to a new eating schedule. But this usually gets better after a little while. Drinking water or herbal teas can help you feel full, and your body will gradually adapt to the new routine.

2. "What if I don't have time to exercise?"

Finding time for exercise can be tough, but there are ways to fit it into a busy schedule. Even short bursts of activity, like a 10-minute walk or a quick set of squats during your break, can add up over the day. Look for small opportunities to move more, like taking the stairs instead of the elevator.

3. "Eating healthy is too expensive."

Eating well doesn't have to break the bank. Buying whole foods like grains, beans, and in-season vegetables can actually be quite affordable. Planning your meals and cooking at home can also help you save money compared to eating out or buying processed foods.

4. "I always end up eating too much at night."

Eating a lot at night is a common habit, especially if you're bored or stressed. Try to find other ways to relax in the evening, like reading or taking a bath. Eating balanced meals throughout the day can also help prevent nighttime cravings.

5. "I'm worried about losing muscle, not just fat."

Losing weight, the right way means focusing on fat loss while trying to keep your muscle. Eating enough protein and doing strength training exercises can help you maintain muscle mass as you lose weight.

6. "I've tried before and failed. How is this time going to be different?"

It's completely normal to try something, and not see the results you hoped for, and have to start again.

Each attempt teaches you something new about what works for you and what doesn't. This time, use what you've learned to adjust your plan, set realistic goals, and maybe find a friend or a group for support.

7. "I don't know how to cook healthy meals."

Cooking healthy meals can seem daunting at first, but it doesn't have to be complicated. There are plenty of simple recipes online that require just a few ingredients. Start small, with easy dishes, and gradually you'll become more confident in the kitchen.

8. "How do I stay motivated?"

Staying motivated can be challenging, especially when progress feels slow. Setting small, achievable goals can help keep you motivated. Also, remember why you started and consider keeping a journal to track your progress and reflect on your journey.

Addressing these concerns involves a mix of practical strategies, patience, and a bit of creativity. Remember, every small step count, and over time, these changes can add up to big improvements in your health and well-being.

Focusing on women over 40 is important because this stage of life brings unique health considerations and challenges. Around this age, many women experience significant changes in their bodies due to perimenopause and menopause. These changes can affect metabolism, weight, bone density, and risk for certain diseases, making it a crucial time to pay extra attention to health and wellness. Here's why it's especially important:

Hormonal Changes

As women approach menopause, levels of key hormones like estrogen and progesterone start to fluctuate and eventually decrease. These hormonal changes can lead to symptoms like hot flashes, sleep disturbances, and mood swings. They can also affect how the body stores fat and manages blood sugar, making it easier to gain weight, especially around the abdomen.

Metabolic Shifts

Around this age, women often notice their metabolism slowing down. This means the body might not burn calories as efficiently as before, making weight management more challenging. A slower metabolism can also impact energy levels, influencing overall activity and fitness.

Increased Health Risks

Women over 40 face an increased risk of developing certain health conditions, including heart disease, osteoporosis, and type 2 diabetes. These risks are influenced by lifestyle factors like diet, exercise, and weight management, making it important to focus on healthy habits during this stage of life.

Muscle Mass Decline

Starting in their 40s, women (and men) begin to lose muscle mass naturally, a condition known as sarcopenia. Since muscle burns more calories than fat, this loss can further slow metabolism. Maintaining muscle through proper nutrition and resistance training becomes crucial.

Nutritional Needs

Nutritional needs can change for women over 40. For instance, they may need more of certain nutrients like calcium and vitamin D to support bone health. Paying attention to these needs can help prevent deficiencies and support overall health.

Lifestyle Adjustments

Focusing on women over 40 is about recognizing the need for adjustments in diet, exercise, and self-care practices to address these changes.

It's about finding sustainable ways to support health, manage weight, and reduce the risk of chronic diseases, all while navigating the challenges of hormonal shifts.

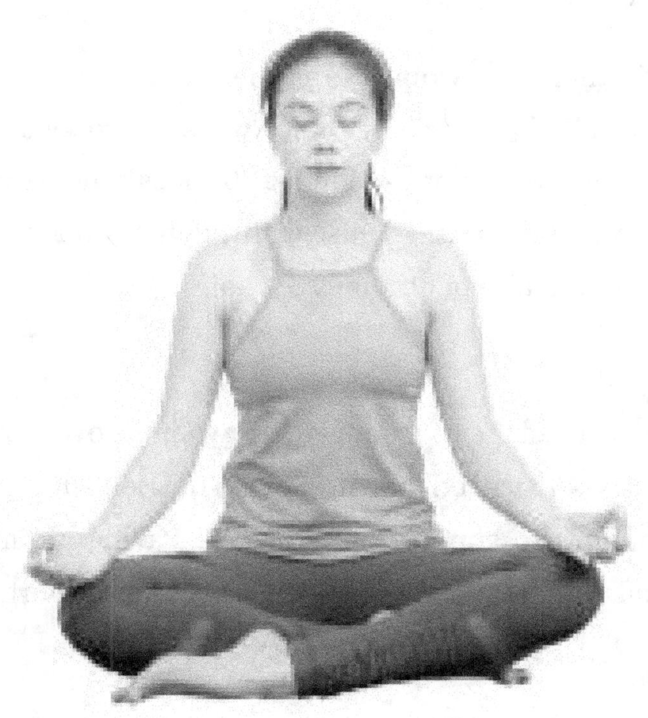

CHAPTER 1:

WHAT IS INTERMITTENT FASTING?

Intermittent fasting (IF) is a way of eating that cycles between periods of eating and not eating. Unlike diets that focus on what you eat, intermittent fasting focuses on when you eat. It's not about cutting out specific foods or food groups but about scheduling your meals in a way that allows your body to spend some time fasting each day or week.

What makes intermittent fasting different from other diets is its simplicity and flexibility. There are no complicated rules about what you can or cannot eat. Instead, the emphasis is on timing. This approach can simplify meal planning and reduce the stress of having to prepare multiple meals or follow strict dietary guidelines.

One of the reasons people like intermittent fasting is because it can fit into a variety of lifestyles. Whether you're a morning person who prefers a big breakfast and an early dinner or someone who isn't hungry until later in the day, there's a fasting schedule that can work for you. Some common intermittent fasting methods include:

The 16/8 method: This involves fasting for 16 hours each day and eating all your meals within an 8-hour window. For example, you might eat between noon and 8 p.m. every day.

The 5:2 diet: With this method, you eat normally for five days of the week and then limit your calorie intake to about 500-600 calories on the other two days.

Eat-Stop-Eat: This involves a 24-hour fast once or twice a week. For example, not eating from dinner one day until dinner the next day.

Intermittent fasting is different because it's adaptable. It doesn't prescribe specific meals or ban particular foods. Instead, it encourages you to listen to your body and eat in a way that supports your natural rhythms. This can lead to a more intuitive relationship with food, where you learn to eat when you're truly hungry rather than out of habit or boredom.

Many people find intermittent fasting helps them manage their weight, improve their energy levels, and even enhance their focus and mental clarity. This could be because fasting periods give your body a break from digesting food, allowing it to focus on other processes like repairing cells and burning stored fat for energy.

It's also believed that intermittent fasting can offer health benefits like improved blood sugar control, reduced inflammation, and better heart health. Some research suggests it might even help extend lifespan, though more studies are needed to fully understand its effects.

However, intermittent fasting isn't for everyone. People with certain health conditions, pregnant or breastfeeding women, and those with a history of eating disorders should consult with a healthcare professional before trying intermittent fasting. It's important to approach fasting in a way that feels nourishing and sustainable, rather than restrictive or punitive.

In short, intermittent fasting is a flexible approach to eating that focuses on when you eat. It offers a simple alternative to traditional diets, potentially supporting weight management and overall health without the need to overhaul what you eat.

A HISTORICAL PERSPECTIVE

Intermittent fasting aligns closely with the evolutionary patterns of human ancestors, who lived as hunter-gatherers for millennia. These early humans didn't have the constant access to food that modern society enjoys.

Instead, they experienced periods of feast and famine, depending on the availability of food. This inconsistency in food availability meant that humans evolved to be metabolically flexible, capable of efficiently using energy from food when it was plentiful and switching to stored fat as a fuel source during times of scarcity.

This adaptability has been crucial for survival and has shaped human physiology to be inherently suited for intermittent fasting.

Cultural and Historical Practices Around the World

Across the globe and throughout history, fasting has been a common practice, integrated into various cultures and religions for spiritual, health, and purification reasons. Here's a look at how different societies have embraced fasting:

Ancient Greece: Philosophers and healers, including Pythagoras, Hippocrates, and Plato, practiced and advocated for fasting as a means to physical health and mental clarity.

Islam: Ramadan, one of the five pillars of Islam, involves a month of fasting from dawn until sunset. This fast is a time for spiritual reflection, self-improvement, and heightened devotion.

Christianity: Fasting is observed in several Christian denominations, most notably during Lent, the 40-day period leading up to Easter. Fasting, alongside prayer and penance, serves as a preparation for Easter.

Judaism: Yom Kippur, the holiest day in the Jewish calendar, includes a 25-hour fasting period dedicated to atonement and repentance. Tisha B'Av and other fast days commemorate significant historical events.

Buddhism: Many Buddhist monks and nuns observe intermittent fasting, refraining from eating after noon until the next morning. This practice is part of a path to enlightenment and detachment from material desires.

Hinduism: Fasting is a frequent and diverse practice within Hinduism, often associated with festivals and religious observances. It's seen as a way to purify the body and mind and express devotion to the gods.

These practices underscore fasting's universal appeal and its integration into the fabric of human culture and spirituality. While the specifics of the fasting practices vary widely across different cultures and religions, the underlying principles of discipline, mindfulness, and purification are remarkably consistent, reflecting a shared human inclination towards periods of dietary restraint for greater physical and spiritual well-being.

The Science Behind Intermittent Fasting for Women Over 40

the science behind intermittent fasting, especially for women over 40. As we age, our bodies undergo various changes, and for women, this period can mark the approach or the beginning of menopause. These changes affect metabolism, hormone levels, and how our bodies process food, making the choice of diet and eating patterns more significant.

Understanding Metabolism

Metabolism refers to how your body converts food into energy. As we get older, our metabolic rate tends to slow down. This slowdown means the body burns fewer calories at rest, which can contribute to weight gain, especially if eating habits remain the same as when we were younger.

Intermittent fasting can influence this dynamic by potentially increasing the metabolic rate slightly during fasting periods. This effect comes from the body needing to tap into stored energy (like fat) to keep functioning, which can, in turn, improve metabolic efficiency.

Hormonal Changes

Women over 40 experience significant hormonal changes, with a decrease in estrogen levels being a hallmark of approaching menopause. These hormonal shifts can impact insulin sensitivity, making it easier for blood sugar levels to become imbalanced, leading to increased fat storage, especially around the abdomen.

Intermittent fasting can help improve insulin sensitivity by giving the body regular breaks from eating. During fasting, insulin levels drop, encouraging the body to use stored fat for energy rather than relying on sugar from food. This process can help manage blood sugar levels and reduce the risk of insulin resistance, a precursor to type 2 diabetes.

AUTOPHAGY

Autophagy is a cellular "clean-up" process that becomes more critical as we age. It involves the breakdown and removal of damaged or malfunctioning cellular components, allowing cells to function more efficiently.

Autophagy is like your body's way of cleaning house. Imagine your cells as little houses where all sorts of processes happen every day. Just like in a real house, waste and broken parts pile up over time. Autophagy is the body's method of taking out the trash and getting rid of these broken parts so everything can keep running smoothly.

Here's how it works: inside your cells, there are tiny structures that act like mini recycling centers. When autophagy happens, these centers wrap up the damaged or unnecessary parts in a little bubble and break them down into basic pieces. Then, your cell can use these pieces to make new parts or get energy. It's a super-efficient way of making sure nothing goes to waste and everything stays in working order.

This process is crucial for reducing inflammation, preventing disease, and promoting longevity.

Fasting stimulates autophagy because when the body is not processing food, it can focus more on repairing and maintaining cells.

For women over 40, enhancing autophagy through intermittent fasting can be a way to support cellular health, potentially slowing down some aspects of the aging process.

Why is autophagy important?

Well, it helps keep your cells healthy, and healthy cells mean a healthy you. By getting rid of the damaged parts, autophagy can protect against diseases, slow down aging, and keep your body's systems running smoothly. It's like maintenance to ensure your cellular houses stay clean, which helps your body function better as a whole.

autophagy plays a crucial role not just in cleaning up cellular debris but also in keeping our bodies running efficiently. This process is like a continuous cycle of renewal within our cells, helping to prevent the buildup of damaged components that could lead to various health issues.

How Does Autophagy Work?

When your body signals that it's time for autophagy, special structures within the cell, called autophagosomes, spring into action. They engulf the damaged or unnecessary cellular parts and then fuse with another part of the cell known as a lysosome.

The lysosome is filled with enzymes that break down the contents of the autophagosome, turning it into basic building blocks that the cell can reuse. This cycle is a critical aspect of cellular housekeeping and maintenance.

Why Is Autophagy Important for Health?

Disease Prevention: By removing damaged parts of the cell, autophagy can help prevent the development of certain diseases, including cancer, neurodegenerative disorders like Alzheimer's and Parkinson's disease, and infections. It's like preventing small problems from turning into big ones by keeping the cellular environment clean and functional.

Aging: Autophagy is also linked to aging. As we get older, the efficiency of autophagy can decrease, leading to the accumulation of cellular damage. This buildup can contribute to the aging process and the development of age-related diseases. By maintaining efficient autophagy, we can potentially slow down aspects of the aging process and extend the health span, the period of life spent in good health.

Immune Response: Autophagy plays a role in the immune system by helping to eliminate invading pathogens and presenting their components to the immune system, which can then mount a targeted response. It's like using the trash to teach the immune system who the bad guys are, so it can better protect the body from infections.

How Can You Support Autophagy?

There are a few lifestyle factors that can help promote autophagy:

Fasting: Periods of fasting have been shown to trigger autophagy. When the body isn't busy digesting food, it can focus more on cellular cleanup. That's one reason intermittent fasting has gained attention for its potential health benefits.

Exercise: Physical activity can also stimulate autophagy. Exercise stresses the cells in a good way, prompting them to start the autophagy process to repair any minor damage and improve cellular function.

Nutrition: Eating a balanced diet rich in nutrients can support the body's natural processes, including autophagy. Some studies suggest that certain compounds found in foods, like spermidine (found in aged cheese, mushrooms, and soy products), can promote autophagy.

Autophagy: A Key to Longevity and Health

autophagy is a critical process that helps keep our cells—and therefore our bodies—healthy by removing damaged and unnecessary parts. It has implications for disease prevention, aging, and immune function. Through lifestyle choices like fasting, exercising, and eating a nutritious diet, we can potentially support this vital cellular process, promoting overall health and longevity.

DETOXIFICATION

Detoxification is like giving your body a good clean-up from the inside. It's all about getting rid of toxins or unwanted substances that you pick up from what you eat, the air you breathe, and even the products you use. Your body is pretty smart and has its own way of doing this clean-up job every day through organs like your liver, kidneys, skin, and even your lungs.

The Role of Fasting in Detoxification

Fasting is thought to support the body's natural detoxification processes, primarily by reducing the intake of new toxins from food and drink and allowing the body to focus its energy on processing and eliminating stored toxins. Here's how fasting may enhance detoxification:

Energy Redistribution: Fasting redirects energy from the digestive system to other systems in the body, including those involved in detoxification, repair, and regeneration.

Autophagy: As mentioned earlier, fasting induces autophagy, a cellular "cleanup" process that can remove damaged and dysfunctional components. While autophagy is more about cellular health than detoxification of external toxins, it contributes to overall cellular efficiency and vitality.

Reduction in Oxidative Stress: Fasting can reduce the metabolic processes that lead to oxidative stress and the production of free radicals, which are harmful substances that can damage cells and tissues.

Enhanced Fat Burning: Since some toxins are stored in fat tissue, fasting-induced lipolysis (the breakdown of fats) may help release and subsequently eliminate these stored toxins.

Considerations for Supporting Natural Detoxification

While the concept of fasting for detoxification is appealing, it's important to approach it with a balanced perspective. The body is equipped with a sophisticated detoxification system that operates efficiently under normal conditions. Supporting this system doesn't necessarily require extreme fasting or detox diets; rather, it can be effectively supported through balanced nutrition, staying hydrated, regular physical activity, and avoiding excessive exposure to toxins.

While fasting offers numerous healing benefits, it's important to approach it with care, especially for individuals with specific health conditions, pregnant or breastfeeding women, and those with a history of eating disorders. Consulting with a healthcare professional before starting any fasting regimen is advisable to ensure it's appropriate and safe for your individual health needs.

How Your Body Detoxes

Liver: Think of your liver as a filter. It spots toxins and breaks them down so your body can easily get rid of them.

Kidneys: Your kidneys are like your body's cleanup crew. They filter your blood all day long, removing toxins and waste in your urine.

Skin: When you sweat, your skin is actually helping to get rid of toxins through your pores.

Lungs: Every time you exhale, your lungs are removing carbon dioxide, which is a waste product of breathing.

Supporting Your Body's Detox System

Even though your body is naturally good at detoxing itself, there are ways you can help it do its job even better:

Stay Hydrated: Drinking plenty of water helps your kidneys flush out toxins. Think of water as helping to keep the river flowing, carrying away waste.

Eat Detox-friendly Foods: Some foods can support your body's natural detox process. Leafy greens, beets, and citrus fruits, for example, can support liver health. Foods high in fiber help keep your digestive system moving, pushing toxins out.

Exercise: Getting active makes you sweat, and sweating helps remove toxins through your skin. Exercise also boosts circulation, helping to move toxins through your body more efficiently.

Get Enough Sleep: When you sleep, your brain actually clears out toxins that have built up during the day. So, catching enough Z's is like hitting the reset button on your body's detox system.

What About Detox Products?

You've probably seen products like detox teas, supplements, or diets advertised as ways to detox your body. While some of these might support healthy habits, it's important to remember that your body is already equipped with everything it needs to detox itself.

Eating well, staying hydrated, exercising, and getting enough sleep are some of the best ways to support your body's natural detox abilities.

In a nutshell, detoxification is your body's way of keeping itself clean and healthy. By taking care of your body with good habits, you can help make sure it's always at its best at getting rid of anything it doesn't need.

When you try intermittent fasting, you're not just changing when you eat; you're also giving your body a special kind of break that can boost its natural cleaning process, or detoxification.

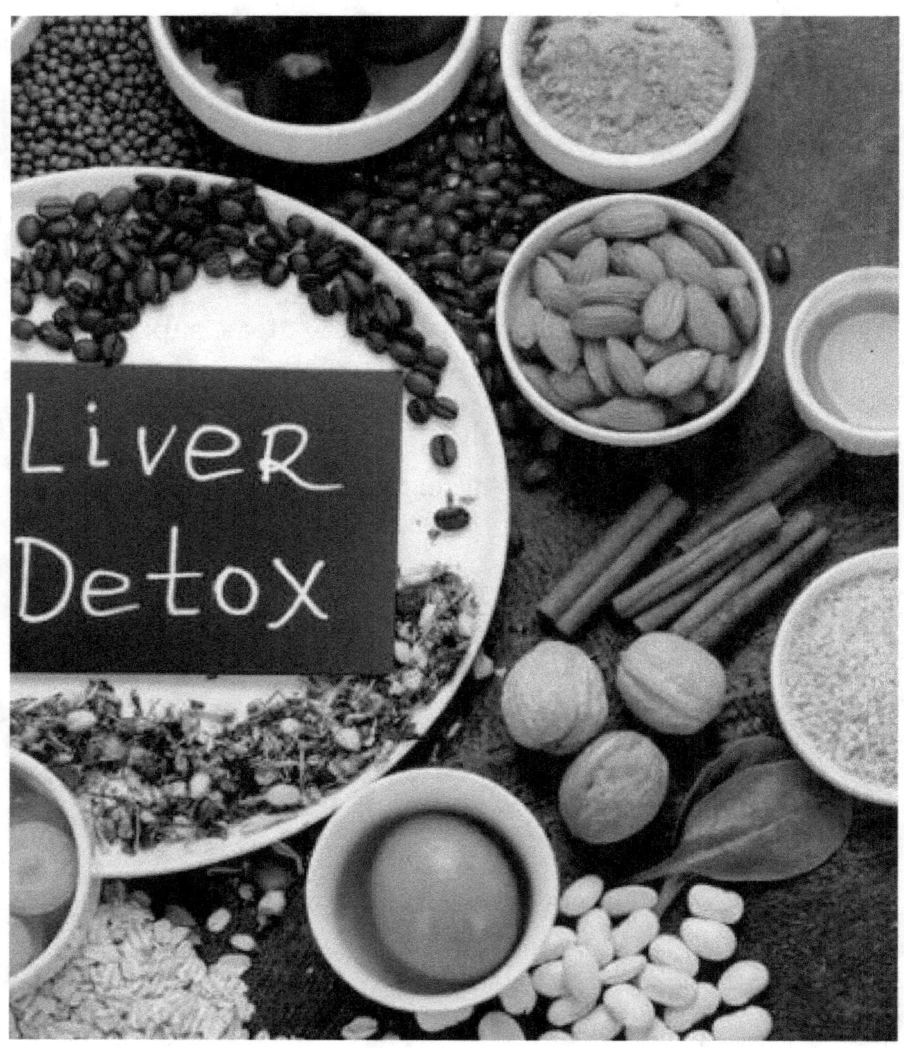

FAT BURNING AND MUSCLE PRESERVATION

Changing body composition is another challenge that often accompanies aging. Maintaining muscle mass becomes more difficult, and fat accumulation, especially visceral fat around the abdomen, becomes more common. Intermittent fasting promotes the use of fat for energy during fasting periods, which can help reduce body fat.

Additionally, when paired with adequate protein intake and resistance training, intermittent fasting can help preserve lean muscle mass. This balance is crucial for keeping the metabolism active and managing weight as we age.

The Impact on Brain Health

Emerging research suggests that intermittent fasting can also have neuroprotective effects. By influencing pathways in the brain related to stress resistance and inflammation, fasting may help support cognitive function and protect against neurological diseases.

For women over 40, this aspect of intermittent fasting could be particularly beneficial in maintaining brain health and function.

In essence, the science behind intermittent fasting for women over 40 involves a complex interplay of metabolic rate, hormonal balance, cellular repair processes, body composition changes, and brain health.

By adapting to and influencing these factors, intermittent fasting can offer a way to support the body through the transitions that occur during this stage of life. However, it's important to approach fasting in a way that's mindful of individual health needs and in consultation with healthcare professionals.

Benefits of Intermittent Fasting for Women Over 40

1. Weight Management and Body Composition

Managing weight and body composition, especially for women over 40, involves understanding how the body stores and uses energy, and making adjustments to diet and lifestyle to support these processes.

The Basics of Weight Management

Weight management boils down to the balance between the calories you consume and the calories your body uses for energy. When you eat more calories than your body needs, it stores the excess as fat. When you eat fewer calories than your body needs, it uses stored fat for energy, leading to weight loss.

The Role of Muscle Mass

Muscle mass is crucial because it burns more calories at rest compared to fat. This means the more muscle you have, the higher your resting metabolic rate. However, as we age, we naturally lose muscle mass, a process called sarcopenia. This can slow down the metabolism, making it easier to gain weight. That's why incorporating strength training into your routine is vital, as it helps maintain muscle mass, supporting a healthier metabolism and better body composition.

Intermittent Fasting and Weight Management

Intermittent fasting can help with weight management by creating periods where your body is more likely to use stored fat for energy. During fasting times, your body lowers insulin levels and increases fat-burning hormones like norepinephrine. This process not only helps with reducing fat but also supports the preservation of muscle mass, especially when you ensure adequate protein intake during your eating periods.

Dietary Considerations

What you eat also plays a significant role in managing weight and body composition. Opting for a diet rich in whole foods, such as vegetables, lean proteins, healthy fats, and whole grains, can support muscle maintenance and fat loss.

These foods provide essential nutrients and help keep you feeling full, making it easier to stick to a healthy eating pattern.

Hydration and Weight Management

Staying well-hydrated is another key aspect of weight management. Sometimes, thirst is mistaken for hunger, leading to unnecessary eating. Drinking enough water can help control hunger, support metabolism, and aid in the breakdown of fats.

Sleep and Stress

Adequate sleep and stress management are often overlooked aspects of weight and body composition. Poor sleep and high stress can lead to hormonal imbalances that increase appetite and cravings for high-calorie foods, contributing to weight gain. Ensuring you get 7-9 hours of sleep per night and employing stress-reduction techniques like meditation or yoga can support your weight management efforts.

Listening to Your Body

Finally, it's important to listen to your body. Everyone's needs are different, and what works for one person may not work for another.

Pay attention to how your body responds to changes in diet, exercise, and lifestyle, and be willing to adjust based on what you observe. Maintaining a healthy weight and body composition is a dynamic process that requires ongoing attention and care.

2. Improved Metabolic Health:

Improving your metabolic health is about making sure all the systems in your body that turn food into energy, and get rid of waste, are working as well as they can. When your metabolism is healthy, your risk for many health issues, like type 2 diabetes and heart disease, goes down. Here's a simple look at how making changes like intermittent fasting can help boost your metabolic health, especially for women over 40.

What is Metabolic Health?

Metabolic health involves a few key things: your blood sugar levels, cholesterol levels, blood pressure, waist circumference, and triglyceride levels (a type of fat in your blood). When these are in the right ranges without using medicines, you're considered metabolically healthy.

How Intermittent Fasting Helps

Intermittent fasting helps improve metabolic health by giving your body breaks from eating. Here's why those breaks can make a big difference:

Better Insulin Sensitivity: Insulin is a hormone that helps your body use sugar from food for energy. When you fast, your body's insulin works better, meaning it doesn't need as much to help manage your blood sugar levels. This is good because high insulin levels all the time can lead to problems like type 2 diabetes.

Lower Blood Sugar: With better insulin sensitivity comes lower blood sugar levels. Keeping your blood sugar stable is key to preventing diabetes and can also help keep your energy levels more steady throughout the day.

Healthier Cholesterol Levels: Fasting can also help change the amounts of different types of cholesterol in your blood, increasing the "good" cholesterol (HDL) and reducing the "bad" cholesterol (LDL) and triglycerides. This helps keep your heart healthy by lowering the risk of heart disease.

Reduced Blood Pressure: Regular fasting periods can lead to a decrease in blood pressure. High blood pressure is a major risk factor for heart disease, so keeping it in check is important for your heart.

Weight Loss and Waist Circumference: Because intermittent fasting can help you lose excess fat, especially around your abdomen, it can decrease your waist circumference. Carrying less weight around your middle lowers your risk for metabolic diseases.

Choose a Fasting Schedule That Works for You: There are different ways to do intermittent fasting, so find a method that fits your lifestyle and that you can stick with.

Eat Nutritious Foods: When you do eat, focus on whole, nutrient-dense foods. Eating lots of vegetables, fruits, whole grains, lean proteins, and healthy fats can support your metabolic health.

Stay Active: Regular physical activity, especially strength training and cardiovascular exercises, can further improve insulin sensitivity and help with weight management.

Monitor Your Progress: Keep an eye on how your body is responding to intermittent fasting. You might want to check in with a healthcare provider to see how fasting is affecting your metabolic health markers.

Improving metabolic health doesn't happen overnight, but with consistent efforts like intermittent fasting, eating well, and staying active, you can make significant strides in boosting your metabolism and reducing your risk for chronic diseases.

3. Enhanced Cellular Repair and Longevity:

As we get older, one of the cool things our bodies can do to help us stay healthy is called cellular repair. This is when our bodies fix or get rid of cells that aren't working right anymore. Doing this can help us live longer and healthier lives. Intermittent fasting, where we switch between times of eating and not eating, can give this process a big boost. Let's break down how this works in simple terms.

What's Cellular Repair?

Think of cellular repair like a cleanup crew for your body's cells. Over time, cells can get damaged from things like stress, pollution, and just normal wear and tear. This damage can make us more likely to get sick or feel old. Our bodies have a way to fix or recycle these damaged cells, called autophagy. It's like our cells are taking out the trash, making sure everything runs smoothly.

How Does Fasting Help?

When you fast, you give your body a break from digesting food, and it can focus more on cleaning and repairing. Here's how:

Boosts Autophagy: Not eating for a while turns up autophagy, helping your body get rid of those damaged cells more efficiently.

It's kind of like doing a deep clean of your house, getting rid of stuff you don't need so everything is tidier and works better.

Reduces Inflammation: Fasting can lower inflammation in your body, which is good because inflammation can make cellular damage worse. It's like putting out small fires before they can spread and cause more damage.

Improves Hormone Balance: Fasting helps balance hormones that are important for growth and repair. For example, levels of human growth hormone go up, which helps with building new cells and tissues.

Longevity

Longevity means living a long life, but it's not just about adding more years. It's about adding more healthy, vibrant years. Research shows that things like autophagy, reduced inflammation, and better hormone balance can all help us stay healthier as we get older. While a lot of this research is still new, and a lot has been done on animals, the signs are promising that intermittent fasting might help us live better lives, not just longer ones.

Tips for Boosting Cellular Repair and Longevity with Fasting

Find a Fasting Schedule That Works for You: There are many ways to do intermittent fasting (like the 16/8 method or the 5:2 diet). Find one that fits your lifestyle.

Eat Well During Eating Times: Focus on foods that are good for you, like vegetables, fruits, whole grains, and lean proteins. These foods can support your body's repair processes.

Stay Active: Regular exercise can also help boost autophagy and improve your overall health.

Listen to Your Body: Everyone's different, so pay attention to how you feel. If a certain fasting schedule isn't working for you, it's okay to try something else.

4. Hormone Regulation and Women's Health:

For women, hormones are like the body's messaging system, telling different parts of the body how to work properly and affecting everything from mood to weight to how well you sleep.

As women age, especially when they hit 40 and beyond, these hormone levels can start to change, which can mess with their health and how they feel day-to-day.

Intermittent fasting, where you cycle between periods of eating and not eating, can play a big role in helping to keep these hormone levels balanced. Let's break this down a bit more.

How Hormones Change

Around the age of 40, many women start to experience shifts in their hormone levels, particularly estrogen and progesterone, because of perimenopause and leading into menopause. These changes can lead to symptoms like hot flashes, weight gain, mood swings, and trouble sleeping. Even insulin, the hormone that helps your body use sugar from food for energy, can start to act differently, making it harder to manage weight and maintain energy levels throughout the day.

How Intermittent Fasting Helps

Intermittent fasting can help manage these hormonal changes in a few ways:

Improves Insulin Sensitivity: When you fast, your body gets a break from processing food, which can help make insulin work better. This means your body is more efficient at using the food you eat for energy, which can help prevent weight gain and energy crashes.

Boosts Human Growth Hormone: Fasting can increase levels of human growth hormone, which helps with metabolism and muscle strength. This can be especially helpful for women over 40, as it can aid in weight management and maintain muscle mass, which often starts to decline with age.

May Help Balance Sex Hormones: While the research is still growing, some studies suggest that intermittent fasting could help balance estrogen and progesterone levels, potentially easing some menopausal symptoms. The idea is that by improving overall health and reducing fat, especially around the abdomen, your body can regulate these hormones more effectively.

Overall Dietary Strategies:

Focus on Whole, Unprocessed Foods: Prioritize fruits, vegetables, whole grains, lean protein sources, and healthy fats. These foods provide essential nutrients for hormone production and overall well-being.

Minimize Processed Foods, Sugars, and Refined Carbs: These can disrupt blood sugar regulation and potentially contribute to hormonal imbalances.

Maintain a Balanced Diet: Aim for a balanced plate with a variety of colors and textures to ensure you're getting a full spectrum of nutrients.

Specific Foods for Hormone Balance:

Cruciferous Vegetables: Broccoli, cauliflower, Brussels sprouts, and cabbage are rich in phytonutrients that support estrogen metabolism and detoxification.

Healthy Fats: Omega-3 fatty acids found in fatty fish, flaxseeds, and walnuts are crucial for hormone production and can help regulate inflammation.

Fiber-Rich Foods: Fruits, vegetables, legumes, and whole grains provide fiber, which helps regulate blood sugar and sex hormone levels.

Protein Sources: Lean protein sources like fish, chicken, eggs, and legumes are essential building blocks for hormones and can promote satiety.

Low-Glycemic Index Fruits: Berries, apples, pears, and grapefruits have a minimal impact on blood sugar and provide essential vitamins, minerals, and antioxidants.

Zinc-Rich Foods: Oysters, pumpkin seeds, and chickpeas are good sources of zinc, a mineral important for healthy ovulation and progesterone production.

Foods Rich in Vitamin D: Fatty fish, eggs, and mushrooms provide vitamin D, which can influence various hormones, including insulin and sex hormones.

Additional Tips:

Consider Including Adaptogenic Herbs: Ashwagandha, maca root, and rhodiola are some herbs with potential benefits for hormone regulation. However, consult a healthcare professional before starting them, as they may interact with medications.

Stay Hydrated: Drinking plenty of water is essential for overall health and can also support hormone function.

5. Cognitive Function and Brain Health:

Keeping your brain sharp and healthy is super important, especially as we get older. Just like the rest of your body, your brain needs the right kind of care to perform its best. This is where something interesting like intermittent fasting can come into play. Let's talk about how taking breaks from eating could actually help your brain.

Boosting Brain Power with Fasting

When you fast, your body goes through a lot of good changes that can also benefit your brain. Here's how:

Ketones: After fasting for a while, your body starts using fat for energy instead of sugar. This process creates molecules called ketones. Ketones are like super fuel for your brain, helping it work better and stay healthy.

Brain-Derived Neurotrophic Factor (BDNF): Fasting increases the levels of a protein in your brain called BDNF. This protein is like a growth booster for your brain cells. It helps make new brain cells and strengthens the ones you already have. Higher levels of BDNF can protect against things like depression and Alzheimer's disease.

Reducing Inflammation: Inflammation in the body can mess with your brain and lead to problems with thinking and memory. Fasting can help lower inflammation, which is good **news for keeping your brain sharp.**

Autophagy: This basically means your cells cleaning up and getting rid of old and damaged parts. Fasting boosts this process in your brain, helping clear out stuff that could make it harder for your brain to work right.

Why It Matters for Your Brain

All these changes from fasting add up to some pretty cool benefits for your brain:

Sharper Thinking: With ketones powering your brain and reduced inflammation, you might find it easier to focus and think clearly.

Better Mood: The increase in BDNF from fasting can also help improve your mood, making you feel more upbeat and resilient.

Long-Term Brain Health: By reducing inflammation and triggering autophagy, fasting could help protect your brain from diseases that tend to show up as we age, like Alzheimer's.

Getting Started

If you're thinking about trying intermittent fasting to help your brain, here are a few tips to keep in mind:

Find a Pattern That Fits: There are lots of ways to do intermittent fasting, from short daily fasts to fasting a couple of days a week. See what fits best with your lifestyle.

Stay Hydrated: Drinking plenty of water is important, especially when you're fasting.

Eat Brain-Boosting Foods: When you do eat, focus on foods that are good for your brain, like fatty fish, nuts, berries, and leafy greens.

INTERMITTENT FASTING AND THE AGING PROCESS

Intermittent fasting (IF) and aging are two topics that have become increasingly connected in discussions about how to maintain health as we get older. IF isn't just about when you eat; it's also about giving your body a break from food, which can have some pretty interesting effects on aging. Let's break down how intermittent fasting might play a role in aging well:

Gives Your Cells a Break

When you fast, you give your cells a chance to focus on repair instead of growth. This break can help clear out damaged parts of cells, a process known as autophagy. Think of it as your body doing some deep cleaning, getting rid of what it doesn't need and making room for new, healthy parts. This can help keep your cells functioning better for longer.

May Help with Healthy Aging

Research suggests that IF could help slow down some aspects of the aging process. By reducing inflammation and stress on cells, intermittent fasting might help keep your body's systems, like your heart and brain, working well as you age.

It's kind of like keeping your car in good shape with regular maintenance, so it runs smoothly for years.

Supports Brain Health

Intermittent fasting has shown promise in supporting brain health and may protect against age-related diseases like Alzheimer's. Fasting increases the production of brain-derived neurotrophic factor (BDNF), a protein that helps brain cells grow and stay healthy. It's as if fasting gives your brain a boost, helping to keep it sharp.

Influences Hormones

Fasting affects hormones that are involved in aging and metabolism. For example, it can increase levels of human growth hormone, which plays a role in growth and metabolism and decreases as we age. Fasting also helps improve insulin sensitivity, which can decline with age, making the body less effective at managing blood sugar levels.

Encourages Weight Management

Maintaining a healthy weight is crucial for aging well, as excess weight can increase the risk of many chronic diseases. IF can help with weight management by limiting the time you have to eat each day, which often naturally leads to consuming fewer calories without the need to count them obsessively.

CHAPTER 2:

IS INTERMITTENT FASTING RIGHT FOR YOU?

Considering Your Health and Lifestyle

Deciding if intermittent fasting (IF) is right for you involves thinking about your health, your daily routine, and what you're comfortable with. It's not just about following a trend; it's about finding what works for your body and your life. **Here's how to consider if IF might fit you:**

Think About Your Health

First up, how's your health? If you have certain conditions like diabetes, low blood pressure, or a history of eating disorders, fasting could complicate these issues.

Women who are pregnant or breastfeeding might need extra nutrients and calories, making fasting not the best idea. Always, the best first step is talking with a doctor or a nutritionist.

They can give you the thumbs up or suggest other ways to reach your health goals.

Consider Your Daily Routine

Are you someone with a super predictable schedule, or does every day look different? Some fasting schedules, like eating all your meals in an 8-hour window, need a bit of planning. If you're juggling a hectic life or your job has you on the go, you might need a fasting plan that's more flexible. The key is finding a rhythm that doesn't make your days harder.

Listen to Your Body

Paying attention to how you feel is super important. Some folks start fasting and feel great: they have more energy, they're not as hungry, and they just feel right. Others might feel tired, grumpy, or just off. If you're giving IF a try and it's not making you feel good, it's okay to reconsider. Your body's feedback is one of the best guides for what's right for you.

Your Goals Matter

What are you hoping to get out of intermittent fasting? If it's weight loss, better focus, or just trying to simplify your eating habits, IF might help. But if your goals are more specific, like gaining muscle or running a marathon, you might need a different approach to food and eating times. Your goals can help guide whether IF is a match for you.

Think About the Long Term

Can you see yourself making intermittent fasting a part of your life for the long haul? The best eating patterns are the ones you can stick with over time, not just for a few weeks or months. If IF feels like something you could realistically keep up, it might be a good fit. But if it feels like a quick fix or too tough to maintain, you might want to explore other options.

Social and Family Life

Consider how IF will fit into your social and family life. Will fasting make meal times with family tricky? What about social outings or work lunches? Sometimes, the challenge with IF isn't the fasting itself but how it fits into your world. Finding a balance is key.

In the end, choosing to try intermittent fasting is a personal decision. It's all about finding what helps you feel your best while fitting into your life in a sustainable, positive way.

ADDRESSING CONCERNS AND MYTHS

Intermittent fasting (IF) has become quite popular, but with that popularity come a lot of myths and misunderstandings. Let's clear up some of these myths:

Myth 1: Intermittent Fasting is Just Another Diet Fad

Truth: While IF might seem trendy, it's based on an eating pattern that humans have naturally followed for centuries, often out of necessity. Recent research supports its benefits for health, weight loss, and longevity, making it more than just a passing trend.

Myth 2: Fasting Means Starving Yourself

Truth: Fasting isn't about starving; it's about scheduling your eating times. During your eating windows, you can (and should) eat nutritious meals to meet your body's needs. The focus is on when to eat, not on severely restricting calories.

Myth 3: Fasting Slows Down Your Metabolism

Truth: Short-term fasting, like the kinds typically done in IF, has been shown to actually boost your metabolism slightly, thanks to increased levels of norepinephrine. However, very long periods of calorie restriction might slow down your metabolism.

Myth 4: You Lose Muscle Mass When You Fast

Truth: If you're doing IF properly and consuming enough protein during your eating windows, you shouldn't lose muscle mass. In fact, IF can lead to less muscle loss compared to traditional calorie-restriction diets, especially if you include some form of resistance training in your routine.

Myth 5: Intermittent Fasting is Bad for Women

Truth: While women do need to approach fasting a bit more carefully due to hormonal sensitivities, many can practice IF successfully. It might involve adjusting fasting lengths and being mindful of the body's cues, especially in relation to menstrual cycles and overall energy levels.

Myth 6: You Can Eat Whatever You Want During Eating Windows

Truth: While IF does offer more flexibility, the quality of your diet still matters. To reap the full benefits of IF, focus on eating balanced, nutrient-dense foods during your eating windows. Junk food can undermine the health benefits of fasting.

Myth 7: Fasting is Impossible with a Busy Lifestyle

Truth: Many find IF fits quite well with a busy schedule since it can mean fewer meals to plan, prepare, and clean up after.

It might take some adjustment to find the fasting schedule that works best for you, but many people report that IF simplifies their daily routine.

Myth 8: Intermittent Fasting Works the Same for Everyone

Truth: Just like any dietary or lifestyle change, individual experiences with IF can vary. Factors like age, sex, health status, and personal goals all play a role in how effective IF will be for you. It's about finding what works best for your body and lifestyle.

Dispelling these myths is important for understanding the true nature and potential benefits of intermittent fasting. As with any change in diet or lifestyle, it's wise to do your research and consider speaking with a healthcare provider to ensure it's a good fit for your individual health needs and goals.

TYPES OF INTERMITTENT FASTING METHODS

Time-Restricted Feeding (16/8, 5:2)

Time-restricted feeding is a popular way to do intermittent fasting, where you eat during a specific window of time each day or week. Let's break down two common methods: the 16/8 method and the 5:2 diet.

16/8 Method

The 16/8 method involves fasting for 16 hours each day and eating all your meals within an 8-hour window. Here's how it works:

Eating Window: You might choose to eat from noon to 8 p.m. That means you skip breakfast, have your first meal at noon, and make sure you finish dinner or any snacks by 8 p.m.

Fasting Window: From 8 p.m. until noon the next day, you don't eat any food. You can drink water, black coffee, or herbal teas during this time to help keep hunger at bay.

This method is popular because it's pretty straightforward and fits well into many people's lifestyles.

It's like extending your overnight fast a little longer, skipping breakfast, and then eating a late lunch and dinner.

5:2 Diet

The 5:2 diet is a bit different. With this approach, you eat normally for five days of the week and then choose two non-consecutive days to eat very few calories. Here's the breakdown:

Normal Eating Days: On five days of the week, you eat your regular meals and snacks, not worrying about restricting calories too much. It's still a good idea to focus on healthy, nutrient-dense foods.

Low-Calorie Days: On the other two days, you drastically reduce your calorie intake to about 500-600 calories for the whole day. For example, you might have a small breakfast and dinner, but keep them very light.

The 5:2 diet can be appealing because you only have to think about fasting or eating very little on two days of the week. It allows for more flexibility on the other days, which some people find easier to stick with.

Eat Stop Eat

"Eat Stop Eat" is a type of intermittent fasting that's pretty straightforward. The idea is simple: you go for a full 24 hours without eating, do this once or twice a week, and eat normally on the other days.

How It Works

Pick a Day: First, you choose a day when you're going to fast. Let's say you decide on Wednesday. You finish your dinner on Tuesday at 7 p.m. Now, your goal is to not eat again until dinner time on Wednesday at 7 p.m. That's your 24-hour fast.

Fasting: During those 24 hours, you don't eat any meals or snacks. But it's important to stay hydrated, so drinking water, black coffee, and tea without sugar or milk is okay.

Eating Days: On the days you're not fasting, just eat like you normally would. There's no need to count calories or change what you usually eat, although focusing on healthy foods is always a good idea.

Repeat: If you want, you can do this twice a week, but make sure your fasting days are not back-to-back. Give your body a break and time to enjoy regular meals.

The Appeal

What makes "Eat Stop Eat" attractive to some people is its simplicity. You don't have to worry about what you're eating all the time or stick to a strict eating schedule every day.

It's just about not eating for a 24-hour period, then going back to your regular eating habits.

The Benefits

"Eat Stop Eat" can help with weight loss because, by fasting, you're naturally reducing your calorie intake for the week. It also gives your digestive system a break, and there's evidence that short-term fasting can boost metabolism and improve insulin sensitivity.

Considerations

Feeling Hungry: Going for 24 hours without eating can be challenging, especially at first. It's normal to feel hungry, but for many, these feelings become less intense as the body adjusts.

Social and Lifestyle Fit: Think about how a 24-hour fast fits into your life. If you've got social dinners or lunch meetings, you'll need to plan your fasting days around these.

Health First: If you have medical conditions or concerns, check with a healthcare professional before trying "Eat Stop Eat" or any fasting method.

Alternate-Day Fasting

Alternate-day fasting is like taking turns: one day you eat, and the next day you fast. It's a straightforward approach to intermittent fasting that alternates between days of normal eating and days of either not eating at all or consuming very few calories. Here's a closer look at how it works and what it involves.

The Basics

Eating Days: On eating days, you eat your meals and snacks as you normally would. There's no need to count calories or restrict what you eat too strictly, but of course, choosing healthy, nutritious foods is always beneficial for your overall health.

Fasting Days: On fasting days, you drastically reduce your calorie intake. Some versions of alternate-day fasting allow for a tiny amount of food, like 500 calories for the whole day, while others recommend not eating at all.

Repeat: You keep alternating between these eating and fasting days. So, if you start with a fasting day on Monday, Tuesday would be an eating day, Wednesday a fasting day, and so on.

Why People Try It

Alternate-day fasting is popular for several reasons:

Simplicity: It's a clear, straightforward pattern to follow. You don't have to think about what you can eat on fasting days since the rules are so simple.

Flexibility: You can adjust which days are your eating or fasting days based on your schedule, making it easier to stick with in the long run.

Potential Health Benefits: Like other forms of intermittent fasting, alternate-day fasting can lead to weight loss, improved metabolic health, and possibly longer life.

Things to Consider

Adjustment Period: Starting alternate-day fasting can be a big change, especially on fasting days when you might feel hungrier than usual. It usually takes time for your body to adjust.

Nutrient Intake: On eating days, it's important to focus on nutrient-dense foods to make sure you're getting the vitamins, minerals, and other nutrients your body needs.

Social and Lifestyle Impact: Fasting days might affect social meals or how you spend time with friends and family. Planning ahead can help manage these situations.

Tips for Success

Stay Hydrated: Drink plenty of water on fasting days to help manage hunger and keep you hydrated.

Be Mindful on Eating Days: While you can eat more freely on eating days, being mindful about your choices can support your goals and health.

Listen to Your Body: Pay attention to how you feel. If alternate-day fasting isn't working for you, it's okay to try a different approach or adjust your fasting plan.

Choosing the Right Intermittent Fasting Plan for You

Choosing the right intermittent fasting (IF) plan for you is a bit like picking out a new outfit—it needs to fit well with your lifestyle and make you feel good. There's no one-size-fits-all when it comes to fasting, so it's important to find a method that matches your schedule and preferences. Let's explore how to pick the perfect IF plan for you.

Consider Your Daily Routine

Think about your typical day. Are you an early bird who loves breakfast, or do you naturally skip it? Do you have a set schedule, or does your day-to-day vary? Some IF plans require eating at consistent times, while others offer more flexibility.

Morning People: If you love breakfast, a plan that allows for an earlier eating window, like 9 a.m. to 5 p.m., might suit you.

Night Owls: If you tend to eat dinner late, an eating window from noon to 8 p.m. could be a better fit.

Look at Your Social and Work Life

Your social activities and work commitments can influence your fasting plan. If you often have lunch meetings or social dinners, you'll want a fasting schedule that accommodates these.

Busy Weekdays: If your work week is packed, starting with a plan that focuses fasting on weekdays might work well, leaving weekends more flexible.

Social Evenings: If you enjoy social dinners, make sure your eating window covers these occasions.

Listen to Your Body

How does your body feel during longer periods without food? Some people thrive on longer fasts, while others do better with shorter fasting periods.

Energy Levels: Notice if fasting makes you feel energized or fatigued. You might need to adjust your eating window or the length of your fasts based on how you feel.

Hunger Signals: If you find yourself overly hungry during fasts, you might want to start with a shorter fasting period and gradually increase as your body adjusts.

Set Your Goals

Your reason for trying IF can also guide your plan choice. Whether it's weight loss, improving energy, or just simplifying your eating routine, different plans might serve different goals better.

Weight Loss: More structured plans like the 16/8 method can help control calorie intake.

Better Health: Plans with longer fasting periods, like 24-hour fasts once or twice a week, may offer deeper metabolic benefits.

If you have diabetes or other health conditions, it's essential to work with a healthcare provider to customize your fasting plan safely.

Start Slow

If you're new to IF, it's okay to start slow. You might begin with a 12-hour fast and gradually increase to a longer fasting period. This allows your body to adjust without feeling too overwhelmed.

Experiment and Adjust

Finding the right IF plan might take some experimentation. Try a method for a few weeks and see how it feels. If it's not quite right, tweak it. The best plan is the one that feels sustainable to you and fits into your life naturally.

Making intermittent fasting (IF) work for you is all about finding a balance that fits into your life smoothly. It shouldn't feel like a struggle; instead, it should feel like a natural part of your daily routine. Here's how to make IF work for you, keeping things simple and straightforward.

1. Pick the Right Plan

Start by choosing a fasting plan that seems like it could easily fit into your schedule. Do you usually skip breakfast? Maybe the 16/8 method is a good starting point. Prefer to eat a bit every day? The 5:2 plan might be better. Remember, the best plan is the one you can stick with without feeling too stressed.

2. Gradually Ease into It

If you're new to IF, don't rush into the strictest plan right away. Begin with shorter fasting periods and gradually extend them. This gives your body time to adjust to the new eating pattern, making it feel more like a natural change than a shock.

3. Listen to Your Body

Pay close attention to how you feel. If you're constantly feeling weak, hungry, or irritable, it might be a sign that you need to adjust your fasting schedule or what you're eating during your meals. Feeling good is a sign that IF is working well for you.

4. Stay Hydrated

Drinking plenty of water is crucial, especially during your fasting periods. Water helps keep hunger at bay and ensures you stay hydrated. You can also enjoy black coffee or tea, which can help make fasting periods easier to manage.

5. Focus on Nutritious Foods

When you do eat, make those meals count by packing them with nutrients. Choose whole foods like vegetables, fruits, lean proteins, and healthy fats. Eating well helps ensure your body gets the nutrients it needs to thrive during fasting times.

6. Be Flexible

Life happens, and there will be times when sticking to your fasting plan is challenging. It's okay to be flexible and adjust your fasting window or even take a break from fasting if needed. The key is to get back to your routine as soon as you can.

7. Use Tools and Support

Consider using apps or joining online communities for support and motivation. These tools can help you track your fasting hours, remind you of your eating windows, and connect you with others on the same journey.

8. Evaluate and Adjust as Needed

After a few weeks, take a step back and assess how IF is working for you. Are you seeing the benefits you hoped for? Do you feel good? If not, don't be afraid to try a different fasting schedule or make adjustments.

Making intermittent fasting work for you is about personalization, patience, and listening to your body. It's not a one-size-fits-all approach, and what works for one person might not work for another. With the right plan, a gradual start, and a focus on nutrition, IF can be a sustainable and beneficial part of your lifestyle.

CHAPTER 3:

PREPARING FOR YOUR FAST: NUTRITIONAL STRATEGIES

Low-Carb Strategies for Ketosis

Getting ready for a fast, especially if you're aiming to enter a state of ketosis, involves some nutritional planning. Ketosis is when your body switches from using carbs for energy to burning fat, producing ketones as a fuel source.

This can not only help with weight loss but may also provide a boost in energy and mental clarity. Here's how you can prepare for your fast with a low-carb strategy to encourage ketosis:

1. Gradually Reduce Carbs

Instead of suddenly cutting out all carbs, try reducing them gradually over a few days before you start fasting. This can help your body adjust more smoothly to using fat for energy. You might start by cutting out sugary snacks and drinks, then reduce grains and starchy vegetables, aiming for a lower daily carb intake.

2. Increase Healthy Fats

As you reduce carbs, up your intake of healthy fats. These are essential for entering ketosis and will become your body's main energy source. Focus on foods like avocados, nuts, seeds, olive oil, and fatty fish. These foods can help keep you feeling satisfied and make the transition into fasting easier.

3. Maintain Moderate Protein Intake

While increasing fats, keep your protein intake moderate. Too much protein can be converted into glucose, which might slow down your entry into ketosis. Aim for a balance with lean proteins like chicken, fish, tofu, and legumes, ensuring you're getting enough to support muscle health without overdoing it.

4. Hydrate Well

Drink plenty of water in the days leading up to your fast. Staying hydrated is key, especially as your body shifts energy sources. Water can also help fill you up and reduce cravings as you reduce your carb intake.

5. Consider Electrolyte Balance

Reducing carbs can lead to a loss of electrolytes, such as sodium, potassium, and magnesium, because your body holds less water without carbs.

To counteract this, consider adding a pinch of salt to your water, eating foods high in these minerals, or taking an electrolyte supplement.

6. Plan Your Last Pre-Fast Meal

Your last meal before starting the fast should be low in carbs, moderate in protein, and high in healthy fats. This can help ease your body into ketosis during the fast. A salad with leafy greens, avocado, nuts, and a protein source, dressed in olive oil, can be a great option.

7. Listen to Your Body

Pay attention to how your body responds to these changes. If you feel overly tired or irritable, you might need to adjust your carb reduction pace or ensure you're getting enough fats and proteins.

8. Be Mindful of Your Goals

Remember, the aim is to support your body's transition into fasting and ketosis, not to deprive or punish yourself. Focus on nourishing your body with high-quality foods that support your energy needs and health goals.

NUTRITIONAL NEEDS FOR WOMEN OVER 40

For women over 40, addressing nutritional needs is crucial for maintaining health, vitality, and a positive quality of life as the body undergoes various changes. This period often coincides with perimenopause and menopause, bringing about hormonal shifts that can affect metabolism, bone density, and cardiovascular health, among other aspects.

1. Calcium and Vitamin D

Why It's Important: Bone density can decrease due to the drop in estrogen levels, increasing the risk of osteoporosis. Calcium and Vitamin D are vital for bone health.

Sources: Dairy products, fortified plant milks, leafy green vegetables, and fish with bones for calcium. Sunlight exposure and foods like fatty fish, egg yolks, and fortified foods for Vitamin D. Supplements may be necessary for some.

2. Iron

Why It's Important: Menstrual changes can lead to increased or decreased blood loss. Iron is crucial for preventing anemia, especially in women experiencing heavy periods.

Sources: Lean meats, seafood, nuts, beans, and fortified cereals. Vitamin C-rich foods can enhance iron absorption.

3. Fiber

Why It's Important: Fiber supports digestive health, helps maintain a healthy weight by providing a feeling of fullness, and can reduce cholesterol levels.

Sources: Whole grains, vegetables, fruits, legumes, and nuts.

4. Omega-3 Fatty Acids

Why It's Important: Omega-3s support heart health, which is crucial as the risk of heart disease rises after menopause. They also benefit cognitive function and joint health.

Sources: Fatty fish like salmon and mackerel, flaxseeds, chia seeds, and walnuts. Supplements like fish oil can also be considered.

5. Protein

Why It's Important: Adequate protein intake supports muscle mass, which tends to decline with age. Protein also plays a role in bone health.

Sources: Lean meats, dairy products, eggs, legumes, and plant-based proteins like tofu and tempeh.

6. Antioxidants

Why It's Important: Antioxidants fight free radicals, reducing oxidative stress and the risk of chronic diseases. They also support skin health as it becomes more prone to dryness and wrinkling.

Sources: Berries, nuts, dark chocolate, green tea, and brightly colored fruits and vegetables.

7. Water

Why It's Important: Hydration is essential for overall health, aiding in digestion, skin health, and the prevention of urinary tract infections, which can become more common after menopause.

Recommendation: Aim for at least 8 glasses of water a day, and consider factors like activity level and climate for adjustments.

8. Vitamins B12 and B6

Why It's Important: B12 absorption can decrease with age, impacting nerve function and energy levels. B6 is important for brain health and mood regulation.

Sources: Meat, fish, poultry, eggs, and dairy for B12. Chickpeas, potatoes, and bananas for B6. Supplements may be beneficial, especially for those on a plant-based diet.

OPTIMIZING HYDRATION DURING FASTING

Staying well-hydrated is key during fasting, as it helps your body function optimally, aids in the removal of toxins, and can even help manage feelings of hunger. Here's how you can optimize your hydration during fasting periods:

1. Start Your Day with Water

Begin your fasting period with a glass of water. This helps kickstart your hydration for the day, especially important if you're fasting overnight and haven't drunk anything for several hours. It's a simple step that can set a positive tone for your hydration habits throughout the day.

2. Spread Out Your Water Intake

Instead of drinking a lot of water all at once, try to spread out your intake throughout the day. Consistent sips can help you stay hydrated without feeling overly full or uncomfortable, especially important when you're not consuming food.

3. Flavor Your Water

If you find plain water a bit boring, consider adding a slice of lemon, lime, cucumber, or a few mint leaves to your water.

This can make it more appealing, encouraging you to drink more throughout the day. Just be mindful of fasting rules if you're following a strict fast that limits any caloric intake.

4. Pay Attention to Signs of Dehydration

Be aware of the signs that might indicate you're not drinking enough water. These can include headaches, dizziness, dry mouth, and dark-colored urine. If you notice any of these signs, increase your water intake.

5. Use Hydration Helpers

Certain herbal teas or black coffee (without sugar or milk) can also help you stay hydrated and can be a nice way to add some variety to your fluid intake during fasting. They can also provide a comforting or warming effect, which can be particularly welcome if you're fasting in cooler weather.

6. Electrolytes Are Important

When you fast, especially for longer periods, your body can lose electrolytes along with water. To help maintain electrolyte balance, consider adding a pinch of salt to your water or drinking a homemade electrolyte drink made from water, a small amount of salt, and lemon juice. This can help prevent electrolyte imbalances.

7. Listen to Your Body

Hydration needs can vary greatly from person to person and can be influenced by many factors, including your activity level and the climate you live in. Listen to your body and adjust your water intake as needed to ensure you're feeling good and staying hydrated.

8. Avoid Dehydrating Beverages

While you might be tempted to drink large amounts of coffee or tea to suppress hunger, be cautious. Caffeine can have a diuretic effect, potentially leading to dehydration if consumed in large quantities. Stick to 1-2 cups and balance it out with plenty of water.

By focusing on staying hydrated during your fast, you can support your body's natural processes, help manage hunger, and enhance your overall fasting experience. Remember, water is a key component of a successful fast, so make hydration a priority.

Importance of Electrolytes

Electrolytes are like the spark plugs of your body. They're minerals that carry an electric charge and are super important for a bunch of things your body does, like moving your muscles, sending signals through your nerves, and keeping your fluids in balance.

The main players in the electrolyte team include sodium, potassium, magnesium, calcium, chloride, phosphate, and bicarbonate.

Why You Need Electrolytes

Fluid Balance: Think of electrolytes as the managers of your body's water levels. Sodium and potassium, for example, help make sure there's the right amount of water inside and outside your cells.

Nerve Function: For your body to send messages from your brain to your muscles and back, you need electrolytes. They help your nerves work the way they should.

Muscle Function: Ever had a muscle cramp? That's your body crying out for electrolytes like calcium, potassium, and sodium which help your muscles contract and relax.

Acid-Base Balance: Electrolytes are also like the peacekeepers that make sure your body's pH level (how acidic or alkaline it is) stays just right.

Blood Pressure: Sodium gets a lot of attention here because it has a big job in controlling your blood pressure.

Spotting an Imbalance

When your electrolytes are out of whack, you might feel tired, get headaches, have muscle cramps, feel sick to your stomach, get confused or irritable, or notice your heartbeat is off. It's your body's way of saying something's not right.

Keeping Electrolytes Balanced

Here's how to make sure your electrolytes stay in harmony, especially when it's hot, you're working out a lot, you're sick, or you're not eating for a while (like when you're fasting):

Stay Hydrated: Drink plenty of fluids. Water is great, but if you're sweating a lot or fasting, you might need something extra to replace lost electrolytes.

Eat Right: Load up on foods that are rich in electrolytes. Bananas and potatoes are great for potassium; nuts and seeds for magnesium; dairy for calcium.

Consider Supplements or Drinks: Sometimes, especially if you're really pushing yourself or not eating, you might need an extra boost from electrolyte supplements or sports drinks. Just watch out for the ones with lots of sugar.

Listen to Your Body: Keep an eye out for those signs of electrolyte imbalance and adjust what you're eating or drinking to help. If things feel really off, it's a good idea to check in with a doctor.

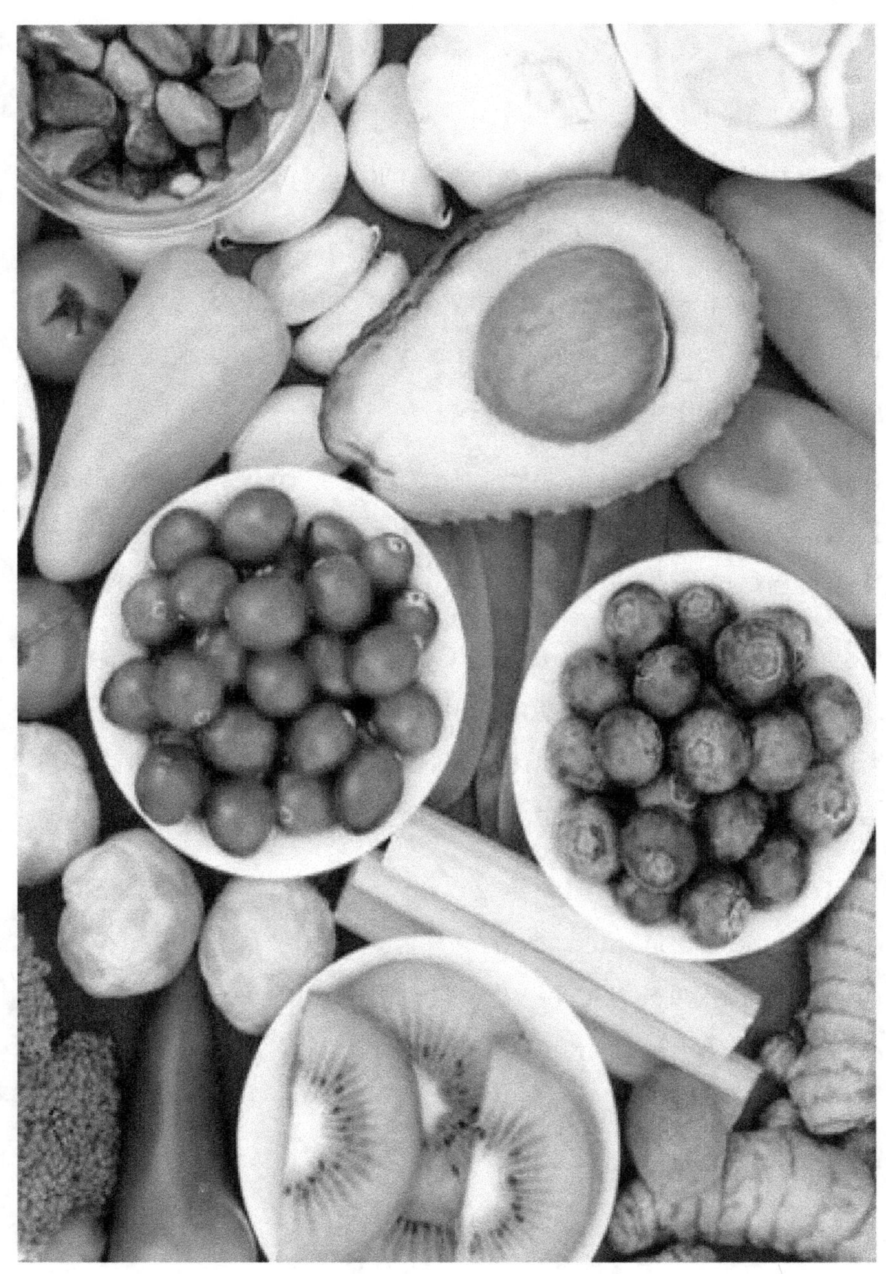

During your eating windows in intermittent fasting, focusing on nutritious, whole foods is key to getting the most out of your fast. However, there are certain foods it's best to avoid or limit, not because they're "bad," but because they might not help you reach your health goals or make you feel your best. Here's a rundown of foods to approach with caution during your eating windows:

Highly Processed Foods

These are foods that come in packages and have a long list of ingredients, often including preservatives, artificial colors, and flavors. They're usually low in nutrients and high in calories, sugars, and unhealthy fats. Examples include chips, cookies, and ready-to-eat meals.

Sugary Beverages

Drinks like soda, sweetened coffee and tea, and fruit juices can be full of added sugars, contributing to a spike in blood sugar levels, followed by a crash. They can add a lot of empty calories without making you feel full.

Refined Grains

Refined grains have been processed, removing the bran and germ, which are the most nutritious parts. This process leaves behind a product that's lower in fiber and nutrients. White bread, pasta, and pastries are examples of foods made with refined grains.

Excessive Fats

While healthy fats are an important part of a balanced diet, consuming too much saturated fat and trans fats can be harmful. These fats are often found in fried foods, baked goods, and some processed snacks, and can increase your risk for heart disease.

Alcohol

Alcohol provides empty calories and can disrupt your sleep patterns and hydration status. If you choose to drink, moderation is key. Also, consider the timing, as drinking alcohol close to your fasting period can make it harder to stick to your fasting goals.

Artificial Sweeteners

Though they're calorie-free, artificial sweeteners can sometimes trigger cravings for more sweet foods and disrupt your body's signals for fullness. Foods and drinks labeled "diet" or "sugar-free" often contain these sweeteners.

DEALING WITH HUNGER PANGS AND CRAVINGS

Handling hunger pangs while practicing intermittent fasting (IF) is a common challenge, but with some smart strategies, you can manage them effectively. Here's how to keep hunger at bay and make fasting periods more comfortable:

1. Stay Hydrated

Drinking plenty of water throughout your fasting window can help reduce hunger pangs. Herbal teas or black coffee (without sugar or milk) are also good options to keep you hydrated and can have a mild appetite-suppressing effect.

2. Keep Busy

Distracting yourself is a great way to forget about hunger. Dive into work, engage in a hobby, exercise, or do anything that keeps your mind off food. Staying occupied not only helps pass the time but also reduces the focus on hunger.

3. Use Mindful Breathing Techniques

Mindfulness and deep-breathing exercises can help manage hunger and cravings. Taking deep breaths and focusing on your breathing can shift your attention away from hunger and reduce stress, which is often a trigger for eating.

4. Plan and Prepare

Don't wait until you're ravenous to eat. Plan healthy meals and snacks beforehand to avoid unhealthy choices when hunger strikes.

5. Break Your Fast with Nutrient-Dense Foods

When it's time to eat, choose foods that are rich in nutrients, fiber, and protein. These foods take longer to digest, helping you feel full longer. Vegetables, lean proteins, whole grains, and healthy fats are excellent choices to include in your first meal after fasting.

6. Gradually Extend Your Fasting Periods

If you're new to IF, start with shorter fasting periods and gradually increase them. This allows your body to adjust slowly, potentially reducing the intensity of hunger pangs as your body becomes accustomed to the new eating schedule.

5. Protein Power:

Ensure you consume enough protein during your eating window. Protein helps regulate hormones that control hunger, keeping you feeling satisfied longer during your fasting period.

6. Consider Electrolyte Supplements

Sometimes, especially during longer fasts, hunger pangs can be a sign of electrolyte imbalance. Adding a pinch of salt to your water or taking an electrolyte supplement (without calories) can help balance electrolytes and reduce hunger.

Cravings

Cravings can be a real challenge, especially when you're trying to stick to a healthy eating plan or following intermittent fasting. They're like little whispers telling you to eat something salty, sweet, or fatty, even when you're not actually hungry. Here's how to deal with cravings in a straightforward and effective way:

Understand Your Cravings

First, it's helpful to understand why you're craving certain foods. Sometimes cravings are your body's way of telling you it needs a particular nutrient. Other times, they're more about emotions, like seeking comfort or stress relief through food.

Stay Hydrated

Believe it or not, sometimes what feels like a craving is just thirst in disguise. Make sure you're drinking plenty of water throughout the day. Herbal teas or flavored sparkling water (without added sugar) can also be satisfying if you're after something with a bit more taste.

Eat Balanced Meals

Filling your meals with a mix of protein, healthy fats, and fiber-rich carbohydrates can help keep cravings at bay. These nutrients help you feel fuller for longer and provide a steady source of energy, which can reduce the urge to snack on less healthy options.

Find Healthy Alternatives

If you're craving chocolate, try a piece of dark chocolate instead of reaching for a candy bar. Want something salty? Opt for a few nuts or seeds. There are often healthier options that can satisfy your craving without derailing your eating plan.

Distract Yourself

Sometimes, the best way to deal with a craving is to distract yourself until it passes. Take a walk, call a friend, or dive into a hobby. Cravings often last only a few minutes, so finding a way to divert your attention can be a powerful strategy.

Practice Mindful Eating

Being mindful about your eating habits can help you understand your cravings better. Before giving in to a craving, take a moment to think about what might be triggering it. Are you really hungry, or are you bored, stressed, or emotional?

Completely denying yourself the foods you love can make cravings worse. It's okay to plan for occasional treats in a way that fits into your overall eating plan. Knowing you have a treat to look forward to can sometimes make it easier to resist immediate cravings.

Get Enough Sleep

Lack of sleep can increase cravings, especially for high-calorie, sugary foods. Make sure you're getting enough rest each night to help manage hunger and cravings during the day.

Managing Social Events and Travel

Navigating social events and travel can be a bit tricky when you're following intermittent fasting, but it doesn't have to derail your progress or stop you from enjoying yourself. Here's how to manage these situations while sticking to your fasting plan, all in a straightforward and stress-free way:

Plan Ahead

Know Your Schedule: If possible, look at your social or travel schedule ahead of time and plan your fasting hours around it. For example, if you have a dinner event, adjust your eating window to fit it in.

Pack Smart Snacks: When traveling, having fasting-friendly snacks (like nuts or seeds) can help you stick to your plan without feeling left out or overly hungry.

Flexibility is Key

Be Flexible with Your Fasting Schedule: It's okay to adjust your fasting hours to accommodate special occasions or travel plans. The beauty of intermittent fasting is its flexibility; you can always return to your regular schedule afterward.

Choose Wisely: When you do eat, opt for healthier choices that are rich in nutrients. Look for meals that include lean proteins, vegetables, and whole grains to keep you satisfied and energized.

Communicate

Share with Friends or Family: If you're comfortable, share your fasting plan with friends or family. Explaining why you're fasting can help them support your choices during social gatherings.

Don't Feel Pressured: Remember, it's your decision to fast, and you don't have to eat just because everyone else is. Politely declining food outside of your eating window is perfectly fine.

Drink Water: Keep a water bottle with you to stay hydrated, especially if you're traveling or at a social event where you might be tempted to eat outside of your window.

Herbal Teas and Black Coffee: These are great options to help you feel like you're partaking in mealtime activities without breaking your fast.

Enjoy Yourself

Focus on the Experience: Social events and travel are about more than just food. Focus on enjoying the company, the conversation, and the new experiences.

Plan Non-Food Activities: If possible, suggest activities that aren't centered around food, like exploring a new place, going for a walk, or playing a game.

Return to Routine

Jump Back In: After the event or trip, return to your regular fasting schedule as soon as you can. Getting back into your routine helps maintain the benefits of intermittent fasting.

Managing social events and travel while intermittent fasting is all about preparation, flexibility, and focusing on the bigger picture.

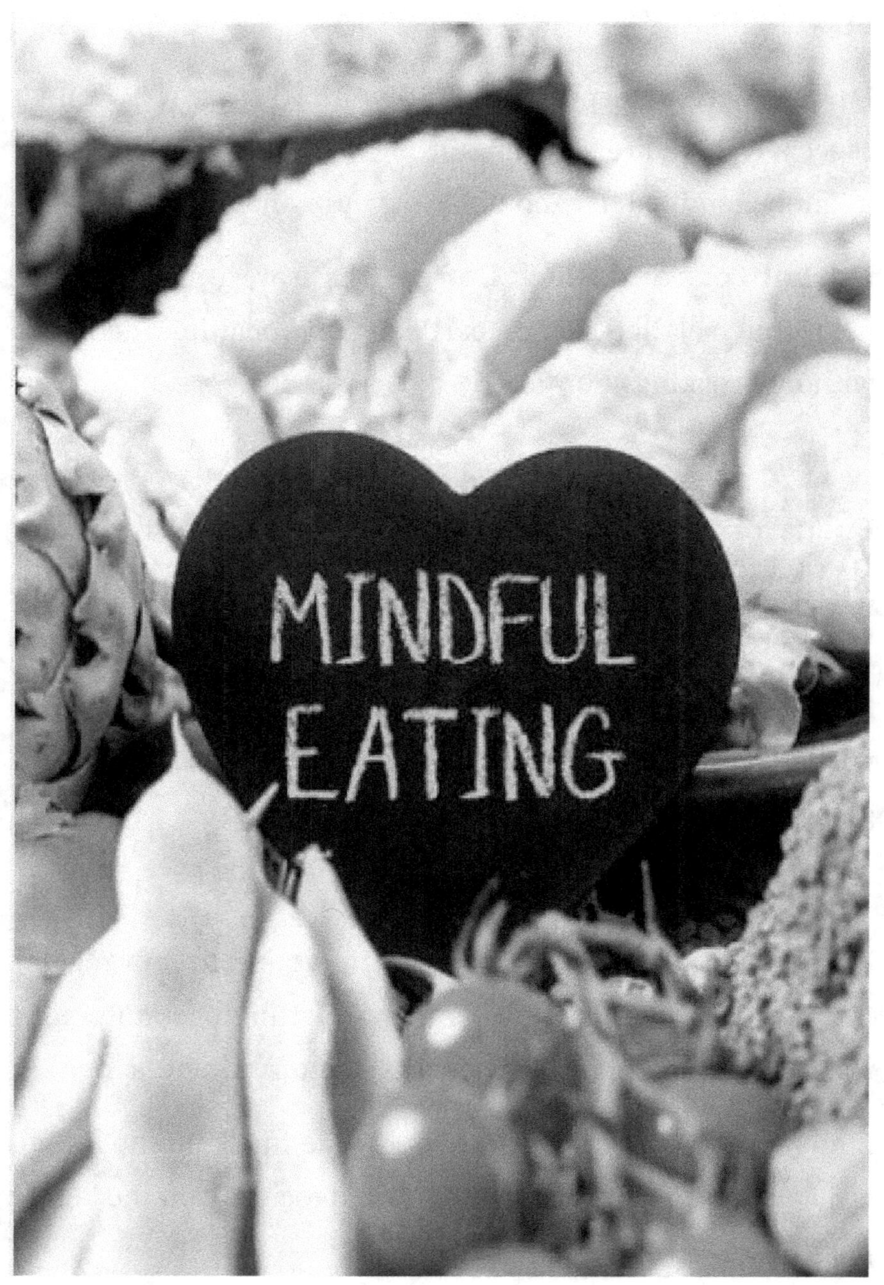

MINDFUL
EATING

CHAPTER 4:

WHAT TO EAT WHEN BREAKING YOUR FAST

Knowing what to eat after a fast is crucial for a smooth transition and to maximize the benefits you've gained. Here's a detailed breakdown on how to break your fast depending on its duration, along with tips for extending it if desired.

Shorter Fasts (14:10, 16:8, 18:6): Gentle Reintroduction

For these time-restricted eating windows, your digestive system hasn't been idle for an extended period. Here's how to gently reintroduce food:

Focus on Whole Foods with Balanced Macronutrients: Prioritize nutrient-rich, whole foods. Avoid sugary drinks and refined carbohydrates that can cause blood sugar spikes.

Excellent Choices for Your First Meal:

Leafy Greens: Spinach, kale, and arugula are packed with vitamins, minerals, and fiber, aiding digestion without overwhelming your system.

Cooked Vegetables: Steamed or roasted vegetables offer essential vitamins, minerals, and antioxidants in an easily digestible form. Choose options like zucchini, carrots, or bell peppers.

Fermented Foods: Yogurt, kimchi, or sauerkraut reintroduce beneficial bacteria to your gut, promoting healthy digestion.

Raw Fruits: Fruits offer a natural source of carbohydrates, vitamins, and minerals to replenish energy levels. Opt for berries or melons for their high-water content and gentle impact.

Nut Butters: Almond butter or peanut butter provide a steady source of energy, healthy fats, and fiber to keep you feeling full and prevent overeating.

Lean Protein: Fish, poultry, or eggs offer high-quality protein to support muscle repair and promote satiety. Choose lean options and avoid fried preparations.

Bone Broth or Soups: The easily digestible protein and soothing properties of bone broth or a light vegetable soup can ease you back into solid foods.

Healthy Fats: Include healthy fats like avocado or olive oil in your meal. These fats provide sustained energy, stabilize blood sugar levels, and aid nutrient absorption.

Portion Control is Key: Avoid a large meal right away, even if you're feeling very hungry. Start with a small meal or a large, balanced snack to prevent digestive discomfort and bloating.

Extended Fasts (24 hours): Take it Slow and Steady

After a longer fast, your digestive system needs even more care when reintroducing food. Here's how to navigate this phase:

Extra Gentle Approach: Be extra mindful when breaking your fast. Your digestive system has been on pause for a longer duration, so prioritize easily digestible options and small portions.

Ideal Choices for Your First Meal:

Bone Broth: This is a classic choice for breaking extended fasts. It's packed with electrolytes, protein, and easily absorbed nutrients, soothing your gut and easing you back into eating.

Cooked Vegetables: Opt for well-cooked vegetables like steamed carrots or asparagus.

These are gentle on your digestive system while providing essential vitamins and minerals.

Easy-to-Digest Protein: Choose easily digestible protein sources like steamed fish or poached chicken. These offer essential nutrients without overwhelming your system.

Foods to Avoid Initially:

Raw Vegetables: Raw vegetables can be taxing on your digestive system after a long fast. Leave them for later in the day.

Beef: Beef is a denser protein source and may be difficult to digest initially.

Fried or Greasy Foods: These foods are heavy and can cause digestive upset. Avoid them until your system is functioning normally again.

Extending Your Fast: Keeping the Hunger at Bay

If you're looking to extend your fast, here are some tips to manage hunger pangs without breaking your fast completely:

Low-Calorie Beverages: Stay hydrated with calorie-free drinks like sparkling water, black coffee, or unsweetened tea. Opt for Earl Grey tea, as some believe the bergamot extract can help suppress appetite.

Mindful Additions (Use Sparingly): If you need a little more to curb hunger, consider these options, but be mindful of their potential impact on the full benefits of fasting:

Bone Broth: Bone broth provides some electrolytes and minerals without a significant calorie count.

Coffee or Tea with MCT Oil or Coconut Oil: These fats may help manage hunger by promoting a feeling of satiety. However, research suggests they might slightly blunt some potential fasting benefits like autophagy (cellular cleanup process).

Supplements to Avoid During Fasting

Avoid certain supplements that can break your fast due to their calorie or carbohydrate content:

Liquid or Gummy Vitamins: These often contain added sugar and calories.

Protein Powders: Protein powders are a concentrated source of protein, typically containing 100 or more calories per serving. They can trigger an insulin response, telling your body it's not in a fasted state.

Branched-Chain Amino Acids (BCAAs): BCAAs are a group of three essential amino acids: leucine, isoleucine, and valine. While they can be beneficial for muscle building and recovery, they can also stimulate insulin production, potentially interrupting the fasted state.

Meal Replacement Shakes: These shakes are designed to be a complete meal in a drink, often containing protein, carbohydrates, healthy fats, vitamins, and minerals. Since they provide a significant amount of calories and nutrients, they will definitely break your fast.

Pre-Workout Supplements: These supplements often contain carbohydrates, caffeine, and other ingredients to boost energy and performance during exercise. The carbohydrates will break your fast, while the other ingredients might disrupt the hormonal changes associated with fasting.

Creatine (with caution): Creatine is a naturally occurring substance found in muscle cells that helps with energy production. While it doesn't necessarily trigger an insulin response, some forms of creatine (like creatine with added sugars) might contain calories that can break your fast. It's best to stick to pure creatine powder if you choose to take it while fasting.

INTERMITTENT FASTING AND HORMONAL BALANCE:

Fasting has emerged as a popular health trend, and for good reason. Beyond weight loss, studies suggest it may positively impact hormone balance, leading to potential health benefits. Let's look into the science behind this connection.

How Fasting Influences Hormones:

Fasting primarily impacts the release and sensitivity of hormones involved in metabolism, blood sugar control, and reproduction. Here's a breakdown of some key hormonal changes:

Insulin: During a fast, insulin levels decrease significantly. This is because your body isn't receiving a constant influx of glucose (sugar) from food. Lower insulin allows your body to access stored energy sources like fat for fuel.

Glucagon: Glucagon, a hormone opposite to insulin, rises during fasting. It signals the liver to release glucose from stored glycogen, maintaining stable blood sugar levels.

Human Growth Hormone (HGH): Studies show fasting can significantly increase HGH levels. HGH promotes cell repair, fat burning, and muscle growth.

Sex Hormones: Fasting, particularly for extended periods, can affect sex hormones like estrogen, testosterone, and progesterone. In men, short-term fasting may slightly decrease testosterone levels, while long-term effects are unclear. For women with excess body fat, fasting can help regulate estrogen levels, potentially reducing the risk of estrogen-dominant health issues. However, prolonged fasting in women with normal weight can disrupt menstrual cycles.

Fasting's Hormonal Effects and Potential Benefits: The hormonal changes triggered by fasting can lead to several potential health benefits:

Improved Blood Sugar Control: Lower insulin levels and increased insulin sensitivity can enhance the body's ability to regulate blood sugar, benefiting those with prediabetes or type 2 diabetes.

Enhanced Fat Burning: Increased reliance on stored fat for fuel during fasting can promote weight loss and improve body composition.

Cellular Repair and Anti-Aging: Elevated HGH levels may stimulate cellular repair processes, potentially contributing to anti-aging effects.

Reduced Inflammation: Fasting may decrease inflammation markers in the body, linked to various chronic diseases.

FASTING AND MENOPAUSE

Menopause, the natural transition when a woman's periods stop, is accompanied by a hormonal rollercoaster. Fasting, a dietary pattern gaining popularity, has shown promise in managing some menopausal symptoms. Let's explore the potential benefits and considerations when combining fasting and menopause.

How Menopause Affects Your Hormones:

During menopause, estrogen and progesterone levels decline significantly. This drop can cause a cascade of symptoms like hot flashes, night sweats, sleep disturbances, weight gain, and mood swings. Additionally, changes in insulin sensitivity and increased inflammation can further impact your health.

Fasting's Potential Benefits During Menopause:

Fasting may offer some relief from menopausal symptoms by influencing key hormones and physiological processes:

Reduced Insulin Resistance: Fasting can improve insulin sensitivity, potentially helping regulate blood sugar levels, a concern for some women in menopause.

Weight Management: Menopause often brings unwanted weight gain. Fasting, by promoting fat burning, may help manage weight and improve body composition.

Inflammation Modulation: Chronic inflammation is linked to various menopausal symptoms. Fasting may decrease inflammatory markers, potentially alleviating discomfort.

Hormonal Shifts: Studies suggest fasting may positively influence hormones like HGH (beneficial for metabolism and cell repair) and sex hormone binding globulin (SHBG), which can help regulate estrogen activity.

Blood Sugar Control: Fasting may improve insulin sensitivity, potentially benefiting women with prediabetes or type 2 diabetes, which are more prevalent after menopause.

Reduced Risk of Chronic Disease: Fasting's potential to improve metabolic health may contribute to a lower risk of chronic diseases like heart disease, which become more concerning with age.

Specific Benefits for Menopausal Symptoms:

Hot Flashes: While research is ongoing, some studies suggest fasting may reduce the frequency and intensity of hot flashes, a common and bothersome symptom.

Sleep Quality: Fasting may improve sleep quality by regulating hormones like melatonin, which can be disrupted during menopause.

Mood Swings: Fasting's potential to reduce inflammation and improve insulin sensitivity might positively affect mood and reduce irritability.

Important Considerations:

While fasting holds promise, it's crucial to approach it cautiously during menopause:

Individualized Approach: Menopausal experiences vary greatly. Consulting a healthcare professional familiar with fasting and menopause is vital to determine the most suitable approach.

Fasting Type and Duration: Different fasting methods exist (time-restricted eating, alternate-day fasting). The optimal duration (16:8, 18:6, or longer) should be tailored to your health and preferences.

Nutrient Adequacy: Fasting shouldn't compromise nutrient intake. Ensure you consume a balanced diet during eating windows to meet your vitamin and mineral needs.

Bone Health: Estrogen decline can increase bone loss risk. During menopause, prioritize calcium, vitamin D, and weight-bearing exercises alongside fasting.

Hydration: Fasting can lead to dehydration. Drink plenty of water throughout the day, even during fasting windows.

Menopausal Stage: Fasting may be more suitable during perimenopause (the years leading up to menopause) or early menopause when hormonal fluctuations are less severe

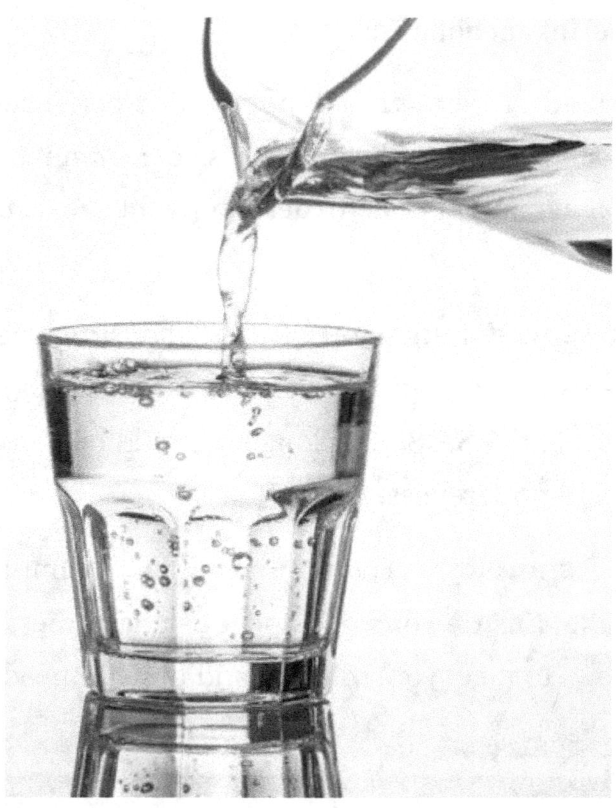

DEALING WITH PLATEAUS

A plateau, in the context of weight loss, fitness, or any personal development journey, refers to a period where progress seems to halt despite continued efforts. After initial success or improvement—whether in losing weight, gaining muscle, improving performance, or acquiring a new skill—there comes a point where no noticeable changes occur.

This can be both frustrating and confusing for many people, as the strategies and routines that previously led to progress no longer seem effective.

Causes of Plateaus

Metabolic Adaptation: As you lose weight, your body requires fewer calories to function than it did at a higher weight. This reduced caloric need can slow down weight loss progress.

Dietary Habits: Sometimes, small changes in eating habits can creep in unnoticed, leading to a higher caloric intake or less nutritious food choices than when you started.

Exercise Adaptation: Your body becomes more efficient at performing the same exercises over time, which means it burns fewer calories doing the same activities.

Underestimating Intake: It's common to underestimate the amount of food being consumed, leading to a smaller calorie deficit than needed for continued weight loss.

Overestimating Burned Calories: Similarly, people often overestimate the number of calories burned through exercise.

Recovery and Stress: Inadequate recovery, overtraining, and high stress levels can affect the body's ability to lose weight and perform, partly due to hormonal imbalances.

Overcoming Plateaus

hitting a plateau means you've reached a point where you don't see progress anymore, even though you're still working hard on your diet and exercise. It's like your body has gotten used to your routine and decided to take a break from changing. Let's break down the tips for getting past this standstill, using a straightforward approach:

1. Eat Just Enough

As you lose weight, your body doesn't need as many calories to keep going. So, you might need to eat a little less to keep losing weight. You can find calculators online or talk to a dietitian to figure out how much you should be eating now.

2. Move More or Differently

To shake things up, try moving more or trying new exercises. If you usually walk, throw in some running or a fitness class. It's about making your body work harder or differently than it's used to.

3. Keep Track of Everything

Sometimes we think we're eating less or moving more than we actually are. Writing down everything you eat and how much you exercise can help you see where you might need to make changes.

4. Change Your Workouts

If you do the same workout all the time, your body gets really good at it, and it doesn't work as hard. Try different workouts to challenge your body in new ways.

5. Sleep and Relax

Not getting enough sleep or feeling stressed all the time can mess with the hormones that control hunger and where your body stores fat. Try to get enough sleep and find ways to relax.

6. Eat Smart

What you eat and when you eat can make a big difference. Eating healthy foods that fill you up without a lot of calories can help, especially if you eat them at times when they can best fuel your body, like before and after workouts.

7. Drink Water

Sometimes when you think you're hungry, you're actually just thirsty. Drinking plenty of water can help prevent this mix-up and is good for your overall health.

8. Try Different Fasting Times

If you're fasting and it's not working anymore, try changing your fasting schedule. Your body might have gotten used to the old one, and shaking things up could help.

9. Take Breaks

Working out too much without giving your body time to recover can actually make it harder to improve. Make sure to take rest days and do things that help your body recover, like stretching or getting a massage.

10. Get Support

Sometimes you just need a little help or someone to talk to. A personal trainer, a fitness group, or a nutritionist can offer support, new ideas, and motivation to get you moving forward again.

Plateaus are just part of the journey. They're a sign that it's time to mix things up a bit. With patience and some changes, you can start making progress again.

CHAPTER 5:

FASTING AND YOUR CYCLE

Aligning fasting windows with the menstrual cycle can be a strategic approach for women to optimize their health and well-being. This concept revolves around understanding the hormonal changes that occur throughout the menstrual cycle and adjusting fasting phases accordingly.

Hormonal Changes:

Throughout the menstrual cycle, women experience fluctuations in estrogen and progesterone levels, which influence metabolic processes and energy utilization. During the follicular phase (days 1-14), estrogen levels rise, promoting fat utilization for energy.

Conversely, during the luteal phase (days 15-28), progesterone levels increase, which may lead to increased insulin sensitivity and a preference for carbohydrate metabolism over fat utilization.

The Power Phase (Days 1-10):

This refers to the days following your period until ovulation.

Estrogen rises during this time, making your body more insulin-sensitive and better equipped to handle longer fasts.

Consider trying 16-24 hour fasts during this window if you feel comfortable.

Focus on low-glycemic index foods when you do eat to maintain stable blood sugar.

The Follicular Phase (Days 11-14):

This short phase follows and leads up to ovulation.

Your energy levels are typically high, and you can likely maintain your fasting routine from the Power Phase.

Feel free to incorporate high-intensity workouts if that's part of your routine.

The Luteal Phase (Days 15-Pre-Period):

Progesterone rises during this phase, leading to a decrease in insulin sensitivity and often lower energy levels.

Shorter fasts (12-hour maximum) are recommended during this time.

Prioritize nutrient-rich foods and focus on complex carbohydrates for sustained energy.

Minimize restriction and prioritize listening to your body's needs.

The Nurture Phase (Week Before Period):

Prioritize nourishing foods and minimize fasting to support your body as it prepares for menstruation.

FASTING A WOMAN'S WAY

"Fasting a Woman's Way" emphasizes tailoring fasting practices to align with the unique hormonal fluctuations and physiological needs of women. Unlike generic fasting approaches, this method recognizes that women's bodies undergo cyclical changes influenced by the menstrual cycle, menopause, and other hormonal factors. Here's an extensive yet straightforward overview of fasting tailored to women:

Understanding Women's Hormonal Cycle:

Women experience hormonal fluctuations throughout the menstrual cycle, characterized by phases such as menstruation, follicular phase, ovulation, and luteal phase. These fluctuations affect metabolism, energy levels, and appetite. Recognizing these changes is crucial for optimizing fasting practices.

Adapting Fasting Practices to the Menstrual Cycle:

Rather than adopting a one-size-fits-all fasting approach, women can benefit from adjusting fasting windows based on where they are in their menstrual cycle. For example, during the follicular phase when estrogen levels rise, the body may be more adept at fat burning, making it an ideal time for longer fasting windows. In contrast, during the luteal phase, when progesterone levels increase, shorter fasting windows may be more suitable to support hormonal balance and prevent potential energy dips.

Embracing Flexibility and Listening to Your Body:

Women's bodies are diverse, and what works for one individual may not work for another. It's essential to embrace flexibility in fasting practices and listen to your body's cues. If you feel excessively fatigued or experience adverse symptoms during fasting, consider adjusting your approach or seeking guidance from a healthcare professional.

Prioritizing Nutrient-Dense Foods:

While fasting, it's crucial to prioritize nutrient-dense foods during eating windows to support overall health and hormonal balance. Focus on incorporating plenty of fruits, vegetables, lean proteins, healthy fats, and whole grains to provide essential nutrients and support optimal functioning.

Addressing Menopausal Changes:

During menopause, women experience a decline in estrogen levels, which can impact metabolism and body composition. Fasting practices can be adapted to support metabolic health during this transition, focusing on maintaining muscle mass, managing weight, and supporting bone health through appropriate nutrition and exercise.

Seeking Support and Guidance:

Embarking on a fasting journey can be challenging, especially when considering the unique needs of women's bodies. Seeking support from a healthcare professional or joining a community of like-minded individuals can provide guidance, accountability, and encouragement throughout the fasting process.

Listening to Your Body:

Above all, it's crucial to listen to your body's signals and honor its needs. If fasting feels overly restrictive or negatively impacts your well-being, it's okay to reassess your approach and make adjustments as needed. Your health and well-being should always be the top priority.

YOUR MENSTRUAL CYCLE

Days 1–10: Low Hormones, Prep for Egg Release

At the start of your period, your hormones—like estrogen, testosterone, and progesterone—are at their lowest. But as your cycle progresses, your body gears up to release an egg. Estrogen starts to increase, making your skin glow and your bones stronger. Plus, it boosts your mood and mental clarity, helping you handle stress better.

Days 11–15: Ovulation Time

This is your prime time! Estrogen and testosterone are at their highest, making you feel powerful and motivated. It's a great time to tackle tasks, start new projects, or crush your workouts. Plus, testosterone helps build muscle, so it's perfect for strength training.

Days 16–18: Hormone Dip

After ovulation, your hormone levels drop, and you might feel a bit low on energy and mental clarity. But don't worry; it's just a natural part of the cycle.

Day 19–Bleed: Progesterone Time

Now it's all about progesterone, the chill-out hormone. It calms you down and prepares your body for a potential pregnancy. But here's the catch: if your stress levels are high, your progesterone might suffer, leading to issues like missed periods or irritability.

Managing Your Fasting Lifestyle:

When it comes to fasting, timing matters. Avoid fasting right before your period, as it can mess with your progesterone levels. Also, remember that progesterone needs glucose to thrive, so don't restrict carbs too much during this time.

Understanding your menstrual cycle and its impact on your body can help you navigate fasting and maintain hormonal balance. So, listen to your body, take it easy when needed, and keep the stress levels in check for a smoother cycle experience.

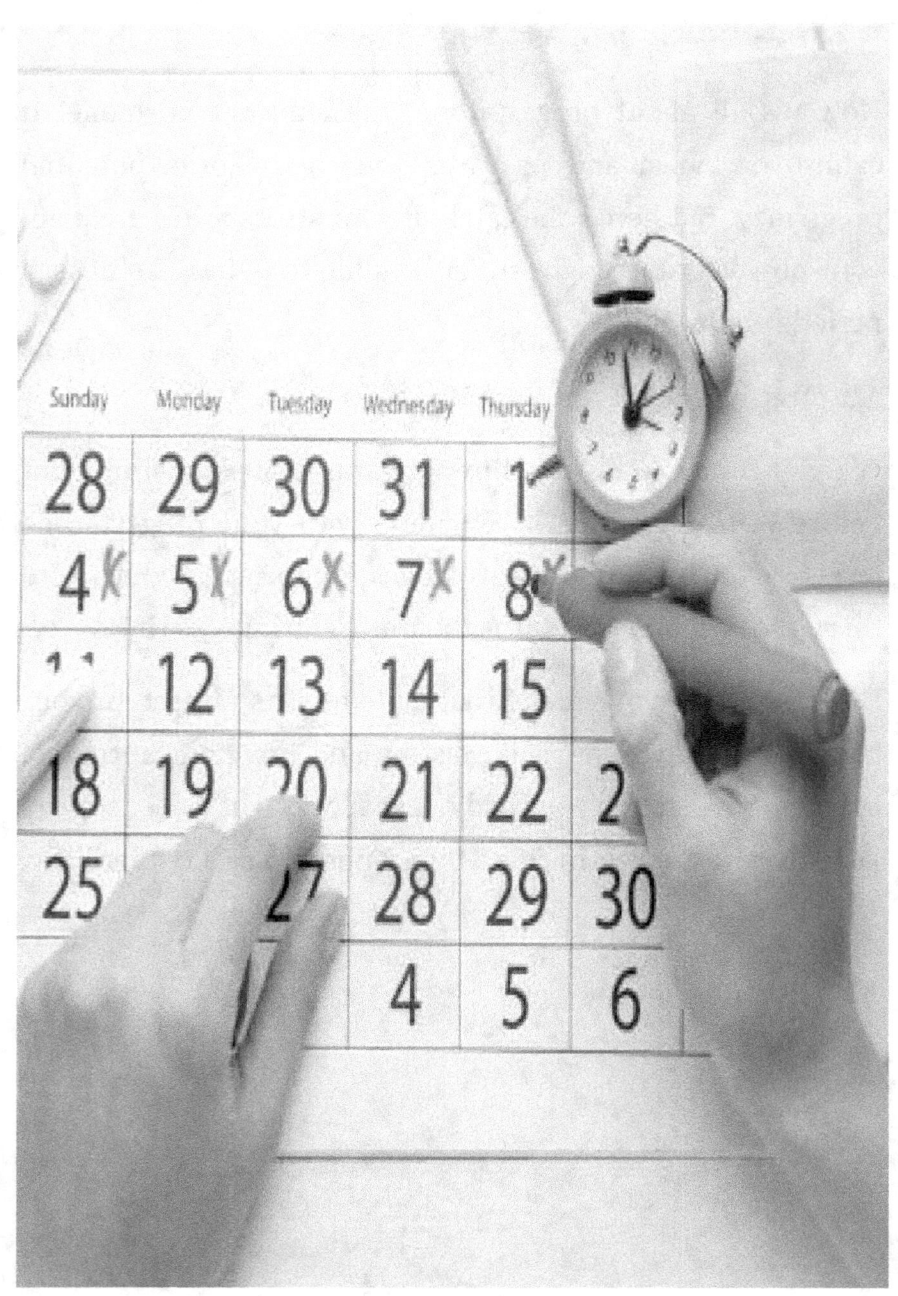

Sunday
Monday
Tuesday
Wednesday
Thursday
28 29 30 31 1
4 5 6 7 8
11 12 13 14 15
18 19 20 21 22 2
25 27 28 29 30
4 5 6

CHAPTER 6:

BREAKFAST RECIPE

Avocado on Whole-Wheat Toast:

Prep Time: 5 minutes: Cooking Time: 5 minutes: Serving Size: 1

Ingredients:

- 1 ripe avocado
- 2 slices of whole-wheat bread
- Salt and pepper to taste

Method of Preparation:

7. Toast the whole-wheat bread slices until golden brown.
8. While the bread is toasting, cut the avocado in half and remove the pit. Scoop out the flesh into a small bowl.
9. Mash the avocado with a fork until smooth or to your desired consistency.
10. Season the mashed avocado with salt and pepper to taste.
11. Once the bread is toasted, spread the mashed avocado evenly onto each slice.
12. Serve immediately.

Nutritional Information (per serving):

Calo: 320: Total Fat: 18g: Fat: 3g: Carb: 34g: Fiber: 13g: Protein: 9g

GREEK YOGURT WITH BERRIES & CHIA SEEDS:

Prep Time: 5 minutes: Cooking Time: 0 minutes: Serving Size: 1

Ingredients:

- 1/2 cup Greek yogurt
- 1/2 cup mixed berries (such as strawberries, blueberries, raspberries)
- 1 tablespoon chia seeds

Method of Preparation:

1. In a serving bowl, add the Greek yogurt.
2. Wash and prepare the berries, then place them on top of the yogurt.
3. Sprinkle chia seeds over the berries.
4. Serve immediately.

Nutritional Information (per serving):

Calories: 200

Total Fat: 7g

Saturated Fat: 1g

Carbohydrates: 25g

Fiber: 10g

Protein: 16g

SCRAMBLED EGGS WITH SPINACH & MUSHROOMS:

Prep Time: 5 minutes: Cooking Time: 10 minutes: Serving Size: 1

Ingredients:

- 2 eggs
- 1/2 cup chopped spinach
- 1/4 cup sliced mushrooms
- Salt and pepper to taste
- 1 teaspoon olive oil or cooking spray

Method of Preparation:

1. Heat olive oil or cooking spray in a non-stick skillet over medium heat.
2. Add sliced mushrooms to the skillet and sauté until they begin to soften.
3. Add chopped spinach to the skillet and cook until wilted.
4. In a bowl, beat the eggs and season with salt and pepper.
5. Pour the beaten eggs into the skillet with the spinach and mushrooms.
6. Stir gently until the eggs are scrambled and fully cooked.
7. Serve hot.

Nutritional Information (per serving):

Calories: 250: Total Fat: 17g: Sat Fat: 4g: Carb: 6g: Fiber: 2g

Protein: 18g

Prep Time: 5 minutes: minutes (overnight soaking required): Serving Size: 1

Ingredients:

- 1/2 cup rolled oats
- 1/2 cup unsweetened almond milk (or any milk of choice)
- 1 tablespoon chia seeds
- 1 tablespoon chopped nuts (such as almonds, walnuts, or pecans)
- 1 tablespoon mixed seeds (such as flaxseeds, pumpkin seeds, or sunflower seeds)
- 1/4 teaspoon vanilla extract (optional)
- 1 teaspoon honey or maple syrup (optional)

Method of Preparation:

1. In a jar or container, combine rolled oats, almond milk, chia seeds, chopped nuts, mixed seeds, vanilla extract (if using), and honey or maple syrup (if using).
2. Stir well to combine all ingredients.
3. Cover the jar or container and refrigerate overnight, or for at least 4 hours.

4. In the morning, give the oats a good stir and add more milk if desired for a creamier consistency.

5. Serve cold and enjoy.

Nutritional Information (per serving):

Calories: 350

Total Fat: 15g

Saturated Fat: 2g

Carbohydrates: 45g

Fiber: 10g

Protein: 12g

COTTAGE CHEESE WITH SLICED PEPPERS & TOMATOES:

Prep Time: 5 minutes: Cooking Time: 0 minutes: Serving Size: 1

Ingredients:

- 1/2 cup cottage cheese
- 1/2 cup sliced bell peppers (any color)
- 1/2 cup cherry tomatoes, halved
- Salt and pepper to taste

Method of Preparation:

1. Place cottage cheese in a bowl or on a plate.

2. Arrange sliced bell peppers and cherry tomatoes around the cottage cheese.

3. Season with salt and pepper to taste.

4. Serve immediately.

Nutritional Information (per serving):

Calories: 200: Total Fat: 6g: Sat Fat: 3g: Carb: 15g: Fiber: 3g: Protein: 22g

SMOOTHIE WITH PROTEIN POWDER & GREENS:

Prep Time: 5 minutes: Cooking Time: 0 minutes: Serving Size: 1

Ingredients:

- 1 scoop of protein powder (flavor of your choice)
- 1 cup of mixed greens (such as spinach, kale)
- 1/2 banana
- 1/2 cup of frozen berries (such as strawberries, blueberries)
- 1 cup of unsweetened almond milk (or liquid of your choice)

Method of Preparation:

1. Place all the ingredients in a blender.

2. Blend until smooth and creamy.

3. Pour into a glass and enjoy immediately.

Nutritional Information (per serving):

Calories: Approx. 250-300: Total Fat: Varies: Carb: Varies: Fiber: Varies: Protein: Varies

BREAKFAST SALAD WITH GRILLED CHICKEN & VEGETABLES:

Prep Time: 10 minutes: Cooking Time: 10 minutes: Serving Size: 1

Ingredients:

- 2 cups of mixed greens (such as lettuce, spinach)
- 4 oz grilled chicken breast, sliced
- 1/2 cup cherry tomatoes, halved
- 1/4 cup cucumber, sliced
- 1/4 cup bell pepper, sliced
- 1/4 cup red onion, thinly sliced
- 1 tablespoon olive oil
- 1 tablespoon balsamic vinegar
- Salt and pepper to taste

Method of Preparation:

1. In a large bowl, toss together the mixed greens, grilled chicken, cherry tomatoes, cucumber, bell pepper, and red onion.
2. Drizzle with olive oil and balsamic vinegar.
3. Season with salt and pepper to taste.
4. Toss until everything is well coated.
5. Serve immediately.

Nutritional Information (per serving):

Calories: Approx. 350-400: Total Fat: Varie: Carb: Varies: Fiber: Varie: Protein: Varies

WHOLE-WHEAT PANCAKES WITH NUT BUTTER & BERRIES:

Prep Time: 10 minutes: Cooking Time: 10 minutes: Serving Size: 1 (2-3 pancakes)

Ingredients:

- 1/2 cup whole-wheat flour
- 1/2 teaspoon baking powder
- Pinch of salt
- 1/2 cup almond milk (or milk of your choice)
- 1 egg
- 1 tablespoon nut butter (such as almond or peanut butter)
- 1/2 cup mixed berries (such as strawberries, blueberries)
- Maple syrup (optional)

Method of Preparation:

1. In a mixing bowl, whisk together the whole-wheat flour, baking powder, and salt.

2. In a separate bowl, whisk together the almond milk and egg.

3. Pour the wet ingredients into the dry ingredients and stir until just combined.

4. Heat a non-stick skillet or griddle over medium heat and lightly grease with cooking spray or oil.

5. Pour about 1/4 cup of batter onto the skillet for each pancake.

6. Cook until bubbles form on the surface of the pancake, then flip and cook until golden brown on the other side.

7. Serve the pancakes topped with nut butter and mixed berries. Optionally, drizzle with maple syrup.

Nutritional Information (per serving, without syrup):

Calories: Approximately 350-400

CHIA SEED PUDDING WITH COCONUT MILK & MANGO:

Prep Time: 5 minutes + chilling time (at least 4 hours or overnight): Cooking Time: 0 minutes: Serving Size: 1

Ingredients:

- 2 tablespoons chia seeds
- 1/2 cup coconut milk
- 1/2 teaspoon vanilla extract (optional)
- 1/2 ripe mango, diced

Method of Preparation:

1. In a bowl or jar, mix the chia seeds, coconut milk, and vanilla extract (if using). Stir well to combine.

2. Cover the bowl or jar and refrigerate for at least 4 hours or overnight to allow the chia seeds to absorb the liquid and form a pudding-like consistency.

3. Once the chia pudding has set, remove it from the refrigerator.

4. Layer the diced mango on top of the chia pudding.

5. Serve chilled and enjoy!

Nutritional Information (per serving):

Calories: 320

Total Fat: 25g

Saturated Fat: 17g

Carbohydrates: 21g

Fiber: 10g

Protein: 6g

HARD-BOILED EGGS WITH EDAMAME:

Prep Time: 5 minutes: Cooking Time: 10-12 minutes: Serving Size: 1

Ingredients:

- 2 hard-boiled eggs
- 1/2 cup edamame beans (shelled)
- Salt and pepper to taste

Method of Preparation:

1. To hard-boil the eggs, place them in a saucepan and cover with cold water. Bring the water to a boil over medium-high heat.

2. Once boiling, reduce the heat to low and simmer for 10-12 minutes.

3. While the eggs are cooking, prepare the edamame beans according to package instructions, typically by boiling or steaming them until tender.

4. Once the eggs are cooked, remove them from the heat, drain the hot water, and transfer the eggs to a bowl of ice water to cool.

5. Once cooled, peel the eggs and slice them in half.

6. Serve the hard-boiled eggs alongside the edamame beans, seasoned with salt and pepper to taste.

Nutritional Information (per serving):

Calories: 240

Total Fat: 13g

Saturated Fat: 3g

Carbohydrates: 11g

Fiber: 5g

Protein: 19g

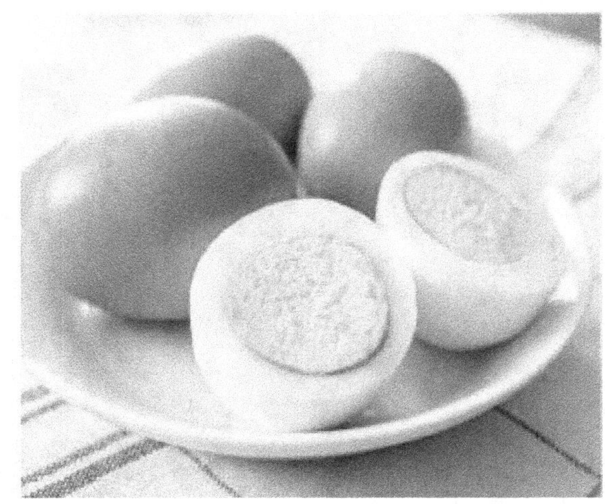

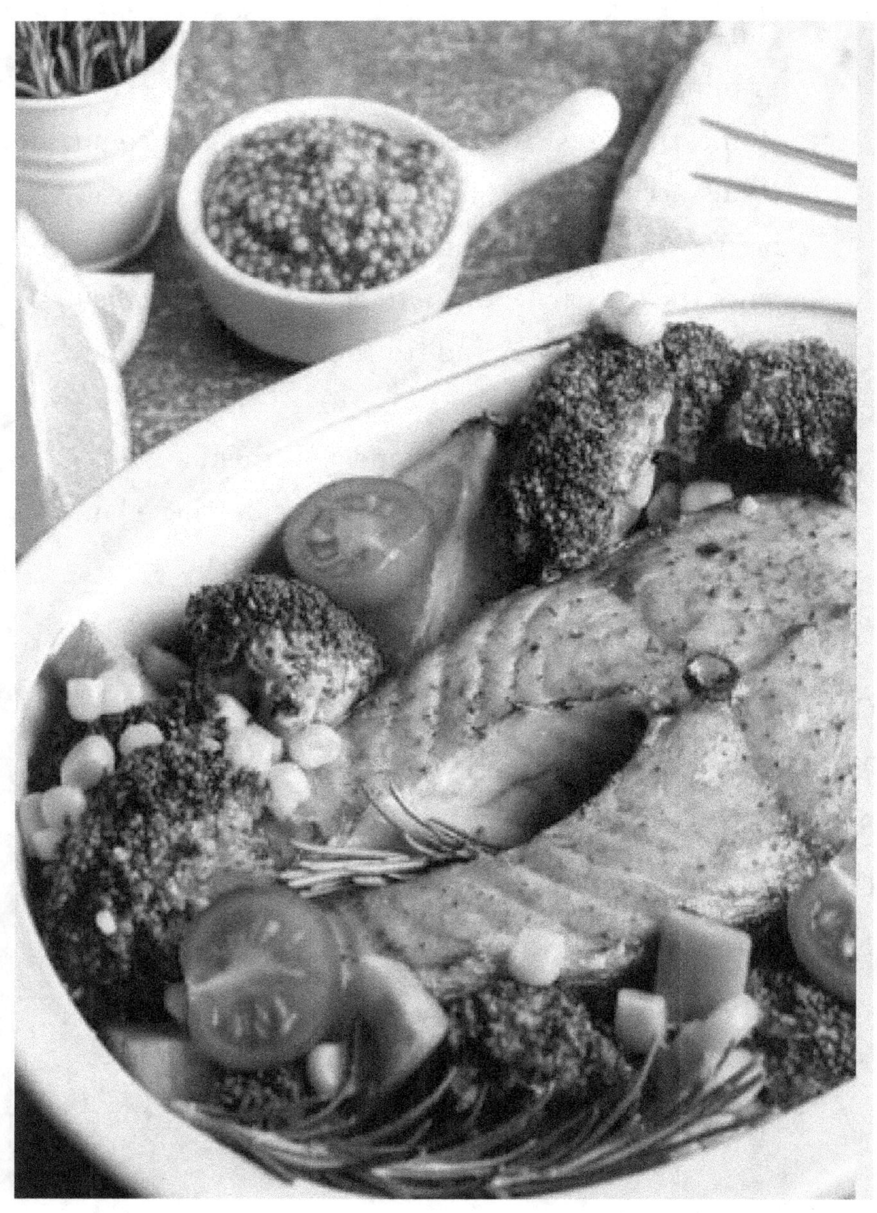

CHAPTER 7:

LUNCH RECIPES

Salmon with Roasted Vegetables:

Prep Time: 15 minutes: Cooking Time: 20 minutes: Serving Size: 1

Ingredients:

- 1 salmon fillet (4-6 oz)
- 1 cup mixed vegetables (such as bell peppers, zucchini, broccoli)
- 1 tablespoon olive oil
- Salt and pepper to taste
- Lemon wedges for serving (optional)

Method of Preparation:

1. Preheat the oven to 400°F (200°C).
2. Line a baking sheet with parchment paper or lightly grease it with olive oil.
3. Wash and chop the mixed vegetables into bite-sized pieces.
4. Place the salmon fillet in the center of the baking sheet and surround it with the mixed vegetables.

5. Drizzle olive oil over the salmon and vegetables, then season with salt and pepper.

6. Gently toss the vegetables to coat them evenly with the oil and seasoning.

7. Place the baking sheet in the preheated oven and bake for 15-20 minutes, or until the salmon is cooked through and the vegetables are tender and lightly browned.

8. Once done, remove from the oven and let it cool slightly.

9. Serve the salmon with roasted vegetables, garnished with lemon wedges if desired.

Nutritional Information (per serving):

Calories: Around 350-400 calories

Protein: Approximately 25-30 grams

Fat: Approximately 20-25 grams

Carbohydrates: Around 10-15 grams

Fiber: Approximately 3-5 grams

TUNA SALAD WITH WHOLE-WHEAT CRACKERS:

Prep Time: 10 minutes: Cooking Time: 0 minutes: Serving Size: 1

Ingredients:

- 1 can (5 oz) tuna in water, drained
- 1/4 cup diced celery
- 1/4 cup diced red onion
- 1 tablespoon diced pickles or relish
- 2 tablespoons mayonnaise (or Greek yogurt for a lighter option)
- Salt and pepper to taste
- Whole-wheat crackers for serving

Method of Preparation:

1. In a mixing bowl, combine the drained tuna, diced celery, diced red onion, and diced pickles or relish.
2. Add mayonnaise (or Greek yogurt) to the bowl and mix until all ingredients are well combined.
3. Season the tuna salad with salt and pepper to taste. Adjust the amount of mayonnaise or Greek yogurt according to your desired consistency.
4. Serve the tuna salad with whole-wheat crackers on the side.

Nutritional Information (approx. per serving):

Calories: Around 300-350 calories

Protein: Approximately 20-25 grams

Fat: Approximately 15-20 grams

Carbohydrates: Around 15-20 grams

Fiber: Approximately 3-5 grams

LENTIL SOUP WITH WHOLE-GRAIN BREAD:

Prep Time: 15 minutes: Cooking Time: 30-40 minutes: Serving Size: 1

Ingredients:

- 1 cup dried lentils, rinsed and drained
- 4 cups vegetable or chicken broth
- 1 onion, chopped
- 2 carrots, chopped
- 2 celery stalks, chopped
- 2 cloves garlic, minced
- 1 teaspoon ground cumin
- 1 teaspoon ground coriander
- 1/2 teaspoon smoked paprika
- Salt and pepper to taste
- Fresh parsley or cilantro for garnish (optional)
- Whole-grain bread slices for serving

Method of Preparation:

1. In a large pot, heat a bit of olive oil over medium heat. Add the chopped onion, carrots, and celery. Cook until the vegetables are softened, about 5-7 minutes.

2. Add the minced garlic, ground cumin, ground coriander, and smoked paprika to the pot. Cook for another minute until fragrant.

3. Stir in the rinsed lentils and vegetable or chicken broth. Bring the mixture to a boil, then reduce the heat to low. Cover and simmer for about 30-40 minutes, or until the lentils are tender.

4. Once the lentils are cooked, season the soup with salt and pepper to taste. You can adjust the consistency of the soup by adding more broth or water if needed.

5. Serve the lentil soup hot, garnished with fresh parsley or cilantro if desired. Enjoy with slices of whole-grain bread on the side.

Nutritional Information (approx. per serving):

Calories: Around 300-350 calories

Protein: Approximately 15-20 grams

Fat: Approximately 5-8 grams

Carbohydrates: Around 50-60 grams

Fiber: Approximately 15-20 grams

Prep Time: 15 minutes: Cooking Time: 15: Serving Size: 1

Ingredients:

- 2 cups chopped romaine lettuce
- 4 oz cooked chicken breast, sliced or shredded
- 1/4 cup grated Parmesan cheese
- 1/4 cup whole-wheat croutons
- Light Caesar dressing (store-bought or homemade)
- Salt and pepper to taste

Method of Preparation:

1. If you haven't already cooked the chicken breast, season it with salt and pepper and cook it using your preferred method (grilling, baking, or pan-searing). Once cooked through, let it cool slightly before slicing or shredding.

2. In a large salad bowl, combine the chopped romaine lettuce and cooked chicken breast.

3. Add the grated Parmesan cheese and whole-wheat croutons to the bowl.

4. Drizzle the salad with light Caesar dressing. Start with a small amount and add more to taste.

5. Toss the salad gently to coat everything evenly with the dressing.

6. Serve the Chicken Caesar Salad immediately, optionally garnishing with additional Parmesan cheese and croutons if desired.

Nutritional Information (approx. per serving, without dressing):

Calories: Around 200-250 calories

Protein: Approximately 25-30 grams

Fat: Approximately 5-8 grams

Carbohydrates: Around 10-15 grams

Fiber: Approximately 3-5 grams

TOFU SCRAMBLE WITH VEGETABLES AND WHOLE-WHEAT TOAST:

Prep Time: 10 minutes: Cooking Time: 10 minutes: Serving Size: 1

Ingredients:

- 1/2 block of firm tofu, crumbled
- 1/2 cup mixed vegetables (such as bell peppers, onions, spinach)
- 1 teaspoon olive oil
- Salt and pepper to taste
- 2 slices of whole-wheat toast

Method of Preparation:

1. Heat olive oil in a skillet over medium heat.
2. Add the mixed vegetables to the skillet and sauté until they start to soften.
3. Add the crumbled tofu to the skillet and cook, stirring occasionally, until heated through.
4. Season the tofu and vegetables with salt and pepper to taste.
5. While the tofu and vegetables are cooking, toast the whole-wheat bread slices until golden brown.
6. Serve the tofu scramble alongside the whole-wheat toast.

Nutritional Information (approx. per serving):

Calories: Around 300-350 calories

Protein: Approximately 15-20 grams

Fat: Approximately 10-15 grams

Carbohydrates: Around 30-35 grams

Fiber: Approximately 7-10 grams

BLACK BEAN BURGERS WITH SWEET POTATO FRIES:

Prep Time: 20 minutes: Cooking Time: 30 minutes: Serving Size: 1

Ingredients:

- For Black Bean Burgers:
- 1 can (15 oz) black beans, drained and rinsed
- 1/2 cup breadcrumbs (whole-wheat if available)
- 1/4 cup diced onion
- 1 clove garlic, minced
- 1 teaspoon ground cumin
- 1 teaspoon chili powder
- Salt and pepper to taste
- Olive oil for cooking
- For Sweet Potato Fries:
- 1 large sweet potato, peeled and cut into fries
- 1 tablespoon olive oil
- Salt and pepper to taste

Method of Preparation:

1. Preheat the oven to 400°F (200°C).
2. In a mixing bowl, mash the black beans with a fork or potato masher until mostly smooth but still a bit chunky.

3. Add breadcrumbs, diced onion, minced garlic, ground cumin, chili powder, salt, and pepper to the mashed black beans. Mix until well combined.

4. Divide the mixture into patties, shaping them into burger-sized rounds.

5. Heat a bit of olive oil in a skillet over medium heat. Cook the black bean burgers for about 4-5 minutes on each side, until golden brown and heated through.

6. While the burgers are cooking, prepare the sweet potato fries. Toss the sweet potato fries with olive oil, salt, and pepper until evenly coated.

7. Spread the sweet potato fries out on a baking sheet lined with parchment paper or aluminum foil.

8. Bake the sweet potato fries in the preheated oven for about 20-25 minutes, flipping halfway through, until crispy and golden brown.

9. Once the black bean burgers and sweet potato fries are done, serve them hot.

Nutritional Information (approx. per serving):

Calories: Around 400-450 calories

Protein: Approximately 15-20 grams

Fat: Approximately 10-15 grams

Carbohydrates: Around 60-70 grams

Fiber: Approximately 12-15 grams

GREEK CHICKEN BOWLS WITH QUINOA AND VEGETABLES:

Prep Time: 15 minutes: Cooking Time: 25 minutes: Serving Size: 1

Ingredients:

- For Greek Chicken:
- 4 oz chicken breast, grilled or cooked, sliced
- 1/2 teaspoon dried oregano
- 1/2 teaspoon garlic powder
- Salt and pepper to taste
- For Quinoa:
- 1/2 cup cooked quinoa
- 1 tablespoon lemon juice
- 1 tablespoon chopped fresh parsley
- For Vegetables:
- 1/2 cup mixed vegetables (such as cucumber, cherry tomatoes, red onion, olives)
- 1/4 cup crumbled feta cheese
- Greek dressing (store-bought or homemade)

Method of Preparation:

1. Season the chicken breast with dried oregano, garlic powder, salt, and pepper. Grill or cook the chicken until fully cooked, then slice it.

2. Cook quinoa according to package instructions. Once cooked, fluff it with a fork and mix in lemon juice and chopped parsley.
3. Prepare the mixed vegetables by chopping cucumber, halving cherry tomatoes, slicing red onion, and pitting olives if necessary.
4. Assemble the bowls by dividing cooked quinoa, sliced grilled chicken, and mixed vegetables among serving bowls.
5. Sprinkle crumbled feta cheese over the bowls.
6. Drizzle Greek dressing over the top or serve it on the side.
7. Optionally, garnish with additional fresh herbs like parsley or oregano.
8. Serve immediately and enjoy!

Nutritional Information (approx. per serving):

Calories: Around 400-450 calories

Protein: Approximately 25-30 grams

Fat: Approximately 10-15 grams

Carbohydrates: Around 40-50 grams

Fiber: Approximately 5-8 grams

TURKEY MEATBALLS WITH MARINARA SAUCE AND ZUCCHINI NOODLES:

Prep Time: 20 minutes: Cooking Time: 25 minutes: Serving Size: 1

Ingredients:

- For Turkey Meatballs:
- 4 oz lean ground turkey
- 1/4 cup breadcrumbs (whole-wheat if available)
- 1/4 cup grated Parmesan cheese
- 1 clove garlic, minced
- 1/2 teaspoon dried oregano
- Salt and pepper to taste
- Olive oil for cooking
- For Marinara Sauce:
- 1 cup marinara sauce (store-bought or homemade)
- For Zucchini Noodles:
- 1 medium zucchini
- Salt and pepper to taste
- Fresh basil leaves for garnish (optional)

Method of Preparation:

1. Preheat the oven to 400°F (200°C).
2. In a mixing bowl, combine ground turkey, breadcrumbs, grated Parmesan cheese, minced garlic,

dried oregano, salt, and pepper. Mix until well combined.

3. Shape the turkey mixture into meatballs, about 1 inch in diameter.

4. Heat a bit of olive oil in an oven-safe skillet over medium heat. Add the turkey meatballs to the skillet and cook for about 2-3 minutes on each side until browned.

5. Transfer the skillet to the preheated oven and bake the meatballs for about 15-20 minutes, or until cooked through.

6. While the meatballs are baking, prepare the zucchini noodles using a spiralizer or vegetable peeler.

7. Heat marinara sauce in a separate saucepan over medium heat until warmed through.

8. In another skillet, heat a bit of olive oil over medium heat. Add the zucchini noodles and sauté for about 2-3 minutes until just tender. Season with salt and pepper to taste.

9. To serve, divide the zucchini noodles among plates, top with turkey meatballs, and spoon marinara sauce over the meatballs.

10. Optionally, garnish with fresh basil leaves.

11. Serve hot and enjoy!

SHRIMP SCAMPI WITH WHOLE-WHEAT PASTA:

Prep Time: 15 minutes: Cooking Time: 15 minutes: Serving Size: 1

Ingredients:

- 4 oz whole-wheat pasta
- 8 large shrimp, peeled and deveined
- 2 tablespoons olive oil
- 3 cloves garlic, minced
- 1/4 teaspoon red pepper flakes (optional)
- 1/4 cup white wine (optional)
- 1 tablespoon lemon juice
- 1 tablespoon chopped fresh parsley
- Salt and pepper to taste

Method of Preparation:

1. Cook the whole-wheat pasta according to the package instructions until al dente. Drain and set aside.
2. While the pasta is cooking, heat olive oil in a large skillet over medium heat.
3. Add minced garlic and red pepper flakes (if using) to the skillet. Sauté for about 1 minute until fragrant.
4. Add the shrimp to the skillet and cook for 2-3 minutes on each side until pink and cooked through.

5. If using white wine, pour it into the skillet and let it simmer for about 1 minute.

6. Add cooked pasta to the skillet with the shrimp.

7. Drizzle lemon juice over the pasta and shrimp. Toss everything together to combine.

8. Season with salt and pepper to taste.

9. Garnish with chopped fresh parsley before serving.

10. Serve hot and enjoy!

Nutritional Information (approx. per serving):

Calories: Around 350-400 calories

Protein: Approximately 20-25 grams

Fat: Approximately 10-15 grams

Carbohydrates: Around 40-45 grams

Fiber: Approximately 5-8 grams

CHICKEN AND VEGGIE WRAPS WITH HUMMUS:

Prep Time: 15 minutes: Cooking Time: 10 minutes: Serving Size: 1

Ingredients:
- 1 large whole wheat or whole grain tortilla
- 4 oz cooked chicken breast, sliced or shredded
- 1/4 cup shredded lettuce or baby spinach
- 1/4 cup shredded carrots
- 1/4 cup diced tomatoes
- 2 tablespoons hummus (store-bought or homemade)
- Salt and pepper to taste

Method of Preparation:

1. Lay the tortilla flat on a clean surface.
2. Spread the hummus evenly over the surface of the tortilla, leaving a small border around the edges.
3. Layer the cooked chicken breast slices or shredded chicken over the hummus.
4. Top the chicken with shredded lettuce or baby spinach, shredded carrots, and diced tomatoes.
5. Season with salt and pepper to taste.
6. Fold the sides of the tortilla in towards the center, then roll it up tightly from the bottom to create a wrap.
7. Cut the wrap in half diagonally if desired.
8. Serve immediately or wrap it tightly in foil or parchment paper for later.
9. Enjoy!

Nutritional Information (approx. per serving):

Calories: Around 300-350 calories

Protein: Approximately 20-25 grams

Fat: Approximately 10-15 grams

Carbohydrates: Around 30-35 grams

Fiber: Approximately 5-8 grams

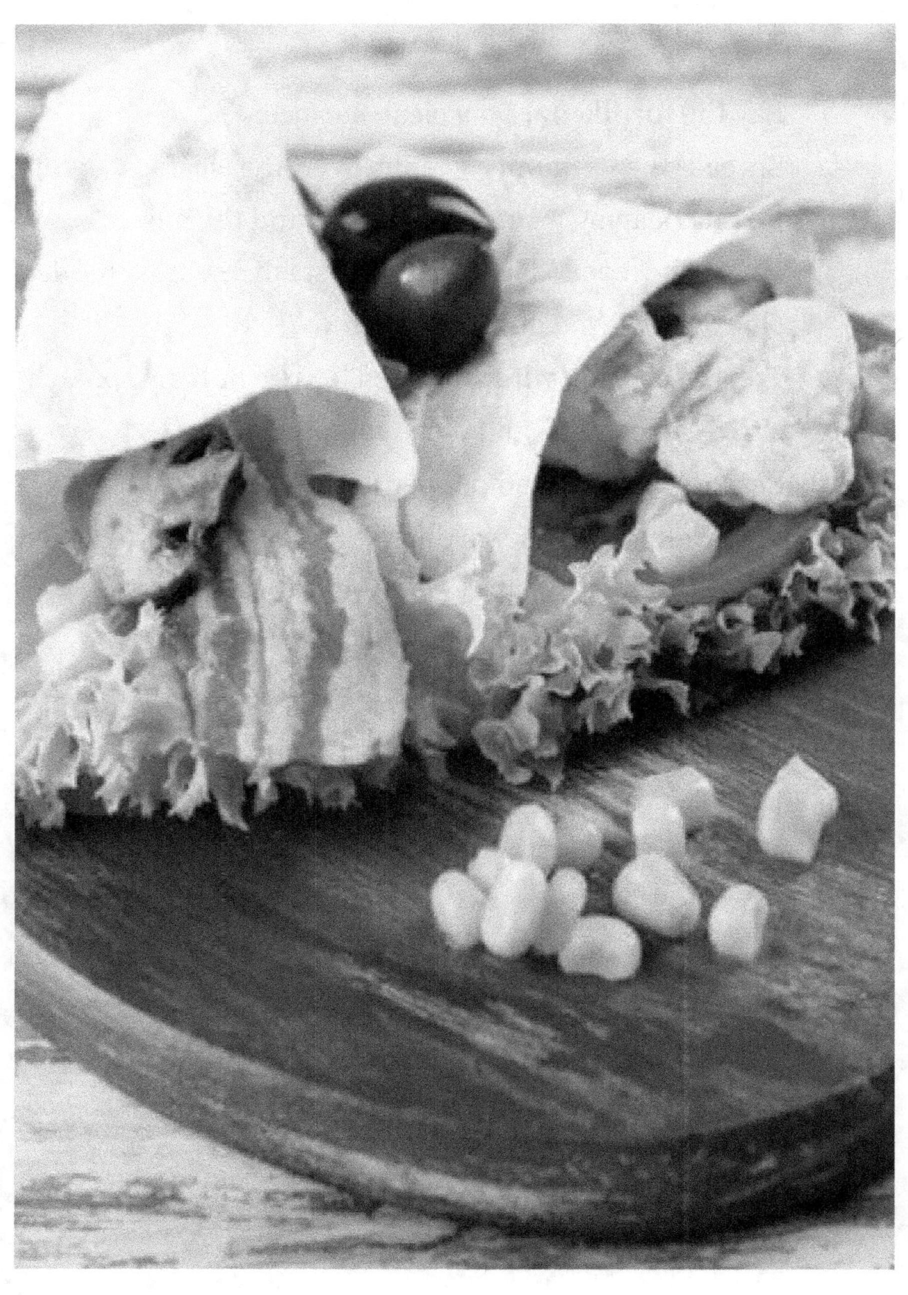

CHAPTER 8

DINNER RECIPES

Shrimp Scampi with Zucchini Noodles:

Prep Time: 15 minutes: Cooking Time: 10 minutes: Serving Size: 1

Ingredients:

- 8 large shrimp, peeled and deveined
- 2 medium zucchinis
- 2 tablespoons olive oil
- 3 cloves garlic, minced
- 1/4 teaspoon red pepper flakes (optional)
- 1 tablespoon lemon juice
- 2 tablespoons chopped fresh parsley
- Salt and pepper to taste

Method of Preparation:

1. Using a spiralizer or vegetable peeler, create zucchini noodles (also known as zoodles) from the zucchinis. Set aside.
2. Heat olive oil in a large skillet over medium heat.
3. Add minced garlic and red pepper flakes (if using) to the skillet. Sauté for about 1 minute until fragrant.

4. Add the shrimp to the skillet and cook for 2-3 minutes on each side until pink and cooked through.

5. Add the zucchini noodles to the skillet and toss with the shrimp and garlic mixture. Cook for 2-3 minutes until the zucchini noodles are just tender.

6. Drizzle lemon juice over the shrimp and zucchini noodles.

7. Season with salt and pepper to taste.

8. Garnish with chopped fresh parsley before serving.

9. Serve hot and enjoy!

Nutritional Information (approx. per serving):

Calories: Around 250-300 calories

Protein: Approximately 15-20 grams

Fat: Approximately 15-20 grams

Carbohydrates: Around 10-15 grams

Fiber: Approximately 3-5 grams

ONE-PAN LEMON GARLIC SHRIMP WITH ASPARAGUS:

Prep Time: 10 minutes: Cooking Time: 10 minutes: Serving Size: 1

Ingredients:

- 8 oz large shrimp, peeled and deveined
- 1 bunch asparagus, trimmed and cut into bite-sized pieces
- 2 tablespoons olive oil
- 3 cloves garlic, minced
- Zest of 1 lemon
- Juice of 1 lemon
- 1/4 teaspoon red pepper flakes (optional)
- Salt and pepper to taste
- Fresh parsley for garnish (optional)

Method of Preparation:

1. In a bowl, combine shrimp, trimmed asparagus, minced garlic, lemon zest, lemon juice, olive oil, red pepper flakes (if using), salt, and pepper. Toss until well-coated.
2. Heat a large skillet over medium heat. Add the shrimp and asparagus mixture to the skillet.

3. Cook for 3-4 minutes, stirring occasionally, until the shrimp start to turn pink and the asparagus is tender-crisp.

4. Continue cooking for another 2-3 minutes until the shrimp are fully cooked and the asparagus is tender.

5. Garnish with fresh parsley if desired.

6. Serve hot, either as is or over rice or quinoa.

Nutritional Information (approx. per serving):

Calories: Around 250-300 calories

Protein: Approximately 25-30 grams

Fat: Approximately 12-15 grams

Carbohydrates: Around 10-15 grams

Fiber: Approximately 4-6 grams

SALMON WITH ROASTED BRUSSELS SPROUTS AND QUINOA:

Prep Time: 10 minutes" Cooking Time: 25 minutes: Serving Size: 1

Ingredients:

- 4 oz salmon fillet
- 1 cup Brussels sprouts, trimmed and halved
- 1/2 cup cooked quinoa
- 1 tablespoon olive oil
- 1/2 teaspoon garlic powder

- 1/2 teaspoon smoked paprika
- Salt and pepper to taste
- Lemon wedges for serving (optional)

Method of Preparation:

1. Preheat the oven to 400°F (200°C).
2. Place the Brussels sprouts on a baking sheet lined with parchment paper. Drizzle with olive oil and sprinkle with garlic powder, smoked paprika, salt, and pepper. Toss to coat evenly.
3. Roast the Brussels sprouts in the preheated oven for 20-25 minutes, or until they are tender and golden brown, stirring halfway through.
4. While the Brussels sprouts are roasting, season the salmon fillet with salt and pepper.
5. Heat a bit of olive oil in a skillet over medium-high heat. Place the salmon fillet skin-side down in the skillet and cook for 3-4 minutes, or until the skin is crispy.
6. Carefully flip the salmon fillet and continue cooking for another 3-4 minutes, or until the salmon is cooked to your desired doneness.
7. Once the Brussels sprouts are done roasting and the salmon is cooked, assemble your meal by placing the cooked quinoa on a plate or bowl, then topping it with

the roasted Brussels sprouts and the cooked salmon fillet.

8. Serve hot, optionally with lemon wedges on the side for squeezing over the salmon.

Nutritional Information (approx. per serving):

Calories: Around 400-450 calories

Protein: Approximately 25-30 grams

Fat: Approximately 20-25 grams

Carbohydrates: Around 25-30 grams

Fiber: Approximately 5-7 grams

CHICKEN STIR-FRY WITH VEGETABLES AND BROWN RICE:

Prep Time: 15 minutes: Cooking Time: 15 minutes: Serving Size: 1

Ingredients:

- 4 oz boneless, skinless chicken breast, sliced into thin strips
- 1 cup mixed vegetables (such as bell peppers, broccoli, carrots, snap peas)
- 1/2 cup cooked brown rice
- 2 tablespoons soy sauce (low-sodium if preferred)
- 1 tablespoon sesame oil
- 2 cloves garlic, minced

- 1 teaspoon grated ginger
- 1/4 teaspoon red pepper flakes (optional)
- 1 tablespoon olive oil or vegetable oil
- Salt and pepper to taste
- Sesame seeds for garnish (optional)
- Sliced green onions for garnish (optional)

Method of Preparation:

1. In a small bowl, mix together soy sauce, sesame oil, minced garlic, grated ginger, and red pepper flakes (if using). Set aside.
2. Heat olive oil or vegetable oil in a large skillet or wok over medium-high heat.
3. Add sliced chicken breast to the skillet and stir-fry for 3-4 minutes, or until the chicken is cooked through and no longer pink.
4. Add mixed vegetables to the skillet and continue stir-frying for another 3-4 minutes, or until the vegetables are tender-crisp.
5. Pour the prepared sauce over the chicken and vegetables in the skillet. Stir well to coat everything evenly with the sauce.
6. Cook for an additional 1-2 minutes, allowing the sauce to thicken slightly.

7. Serve the chicken stir-fry over cooked brown rice.

8. Garnish with sesame seeds and sliced green onions if desired.

9. Enjoy hot!

Nutritional Information (approx. per serving):

Calories: Around 350-400 calories

Protein: Approximately 25-30 grams

Fat: Approximately 10-15 grams

Carbohydrates: Around 30-35 grams

Fiber: Approximately 5-7 grams

LENTIL SHEPHERD'S PIE WITH MASHED CAULIFLOWER:

Prep Time: 20 minutes: Cooking Time: 40 minutes: Serving Size: 1

Ingredients:

- 1 cup dry green or brown lentils
- 2 cups vegetable broth
- 1 onion, diced
- 2 carrots, diced
- 2 celery stalks, diced
- 2 cloves garlic, minced
- 1 tablespoon tomato paste
- 1 teaspoon dried thyme

- 1 teaspoon dried rosemary

- Salt and pepper to taste

- 1 head cauliflower, chopped into florets

- 2 tablespoons unsweetened almond milk (or any milk of your choice)

- 1 tablespoon olive oil

- Paprika for garnish (optional)

Method of Preparation:

1. Rinse the lentils under cold water and drain.

2. In a large pot, combine the lentils and vegetable broth. Bring to a boil, then reduce heat to simmer and cook for 20-25 minutes, or until lentils are tender but not mushy. Drain any excess liquid.

3. In another large skillet, heat olive oil over medium heat. Add diced onion, carrots, and celery. Cook until vegetables are softened, about 5-7 minutes.

4. Add minced garlic, tomato paste, dried thyme, dried rosemary, salt, and pepper to the skillet. Cook for another 1-2 minutes, until fragrant.

5. Preheat the oven to 375°F (190°C).

6. Transfer the cooked lentils to the skillet with the vegetables. Stir to combine and cook for an additional 2-3 minutes.

7. While the lentil mixture is cooking, steam the cauliflower florets until very tender, about 10-15 minutes.

8. Once the cauliflower is cooked, transfer it to a food processor. Add almond milk, salt, and pepper to taste. Blend until smooth and creamy, resembling mashed potatoes.

9. Transfer the lentil mixture to a baking dish. Spread the mashed cauliflower evenly over the top.

10. Sprinkle with paprika for garnish if desired.

11. Bake in the preheated oven for 15-20 minutes, or until the top is lightly golden and the filling is bubbly.

12. Let cool slightly before serving.

13. Enjoy your Lentil Shepherd's Pie with Mashed Cauliflower hot!

Nutritional Information (approx. per serving):

Calories: Around 300-350 calories

Protein: Approximately 15-20 grams

Fat: Approximately 5-10 grams

Carbohydrates: Around 50-60 grams

Fiber: Approximately 15-20 grams

BAKED TOFU WITH SPICY PEANUT SAUCE AND BROCCOLI:

Prep Time: 15 minutes: Cooking Time: 25 minutes: Serving Size: 1

Ingredients:

- 1 block (about 14 oz) firm tofu, pressed and cut into cubes
- 2 cups broccoli florets
- 2 tablespoons soy sauce (or tamari for gluten-free option)
- 2 tablespoons peanut butter (smooth or crunchy)
- 1 tablespoon maple syrup or honey
- 1 tablespoon rice vinegar
- 1 tablespoon sriracha sauce (adjust to taste for desired spiciness)
- 1 clove garlic, minced
- 1 teaspoon grated ginger
- 1 tablespoon sesame oil
- 2 tablespoons water
- Sesame seeds and chopped green onions for garnish (optional)

Method of Preparation:

1. Preheat the oven to 400°F (200°C).

2. In a small bowl, whisk together soy sauce, peanut butter, maple syrup or honey, rice vinegar, sriracha sauce, minced garlic, grated ginger, sesame oil, and water to make the spicy peanut sauce.

3. Place the tofu cubes in a single layer on a baking sheet lined with parchment paper or lightly greased.

4. Pour half of the spicy peanut sauce over the tofu cubes, reserving the other half for later. Toss to coat the tofu evenly.

5. Arrange the broccoli florets around the tofu on the baking sheet.

6. Bake in the preheated oven for 20-25 minutes, or until the tofu is golden and crispy, and the broccoli is tender-crisp.

7. Remove from the oven and drizzle the remaining spicy peanut sauce over the baked tofu and broccoli.

8. Garnish with sesame seeds and chopped green onions if desired.

9. Serve hot and enjoy!

Nutritional Information (approx. per serving):
Calories: Around 300-350 calories

Protein: Approximately 15-20 grams

Fat: Approximately 15-20 grams

Carbohydrates: Around 20-25 grams

Fiber: Approximately 5-8 grams

BLACK BEAN AND QUINOA STUFFED PEPPERS:

Prep Time: 15 minutes: Cooking Time: 40 minutes: Serving Size: 1 stuffed pepper

Ingredients:

- 4 large bell peppers, any color
- 1 cup cooked quinoa
- 1 can (15 oz) black beans, drained and rinsed
- 1 cup diced tomatoes
- 1 cup corn kernels (fresh, canned, or frozen)
- 1/2 cup diced onion
- 2 cloves garlic, minced
- 1 teaspoon chili powder
- 1 teaspoon cumin
- Salt and pepper to taste
- 1/2 cup shredded cheese (optional, for topping)
- Fresh cilantro or parsley for garnish (optional)

Method of Preparation:

1. Preheat the oven to 375°F (190°C).
2. Cut the tops off the bell peppers and remove the seeds and membranes from the inside. Rinse them under cold water and pat dry with paper towels.

3. In a large mixing bowl, combine cooked quinoa, black beans, diced tomatoes, corn kernels, diced onion, minced garlic, chili powder, cumin, salt, and pepper. Mix well to combine.

4. Spoon the quinoa and black bean mixture evenly into each bell pepper, pressing down gently to pack the filling.

5. Place the stuffed peppers upright in a baking dish.

6. Cover the baking dish with aluminum foil and bake in the preheated oven for 30 minutes.

7. After 30 minutes, remove the foil from the baking dish. If using shredded cheese, sprinkle it over the top of each stuffed pepper.

8. Return the baking dish to the oven, uncovered, and bake for an additional 10 minutes, or until the peppers are tender and the cheese is melted and bubbly.

9. Remove from the oven and let the stuffed peppers cool for a few minutes before serving.

10. Garnish with fresh cilantro or parsley if desired.

11. Serve hot and enjoy!

Nutritional Info (approx. per stuffed pepper):

Calories: Around 250-300 calories: Protein: Approx. 10-15 grams: Fat: Approx. 5-8 grams: Carbohydrates: Around 40-45 grams: Fiber: Approximately 10-15 grams

Prep Time: 15 minutes: Cooking Time: 25 minutes: Serving Size: 1 cup

Ingredients:

- 8 oz whole-wheat egg noodles
- 2 cans (5 oz each) tuna, drained
- 1 cup frozen peas, thawed
- 1 cup sliced mushrooms
- 1/2 cup diced onion
- 2 cloves garlic, minced
- 2 tablespoons butter or olive oil
- 2 tablespoons all-purpose flour
- 1 1/2 cups milk
- 1/2 cup shredded cheddar cheese
- Salt and pepper to taste
- 1/2 cup breadcrumbs (whole-wheat if available)
- Fresh parsley for garnish (optional)

Method of Preparation:

1. Preheat the oven to 375°F (190°C). Grease a 9x13-inch baking dish.
2. Cook the whole-wheat egg noodles according to the package instructions until al dente. Drain and set aside.

3. In a large skillet, heat butter or olive oil over medium heat. Add diced onion and sliced mushrooms. Cook until softened, about 5 minutes.

4. Add minced garlic to the skillet and cook for another minute until fragrant.

5. Sprinkle flour over the vegetables in the skillet and stir to coat evenly. Cook for 1-2 minutes to cook off the raw flour taste.

6. Gradually pour in milk while stirring continuously to avoid lumps. Cook until the sauce thickens, about 3-5 minutes.

7. Stir in shredded cheddar cheese until melted and smooth. Season with salt and pepper to taste.

8. Add drained tuna and thawed peas to the skillet. Stir to combine.

9. Add the cooked whole-wheat egg noodles to the skillet and toss everything together until well mixed.

10. Transfer the tuna noodle mixture to the greased baking dish. Spread it out evenly.

11. Sprinkle breadcrumbs over the top of the casserole.

12. Bake in the preheated oven for 20-25 minutes, or until the top is golden brown and the casserole is bubbly.

13. Remove from the oven and let it cool for a few minutes before serving.

14. Garnish with fresh parsley if desired.

15. Serve hot and enjoy!

Nutritional Information (approx. per serving):

Calories: Around 350-400 calories

Protein: Approximately 25-30 grams

Fat: Approximately 10-15 grams

Carbohydrates: Around 40-45 grams

Fiber: Approximately 5-8 grams

GREEK YOGURT BOWLS WITH CHICKEN, VEGETABLES, AND TZATZIKI SAUCE:

Prep Time: 20 minutes: Cooking Time: 20 minutes: Serving Size: 1 bowl

Ingredients:

- 4 oz boneless, skinless chicken breast, sliced into strips
- 1 cup Greek yogurt (plain, unsweetened)
- 1 cucumber, grated
- 1/2 cup cherry tomatoes, halved
- 1/4 cup sliced red onion
- 1/4 cup sliced bell peppers (any color)
- 2 tablespoons fresh lemon juice
- 2 cloves garlic, minced
- 1 tablespoon chopped fresh dill
- Salt and pepper to taste

- Olive oil for cooking
- For Tzatziki Sauce:
- 1/2 cup Greek yogurt (plain, unsweetened)
- 1/2 cucumber, grated and drained
- 1 clove garlic, minced
- 1 tablespoon fresh lemon juice
- 1 tablespoon chopped fresh dill
- Salt and pepper to taste

Method of Preparation:

1. In a bowl, combine 1 cup of Greek yogurt with grated cucumber, minced garlic, chopped dill, lemon juice, salt, and pepper to make the tzatziki sauce. Mix well and set aside.

2. Heat olive oil in a skillet over medium-high heat. Add sliced chicken breast strips to the skillet and cook until golden brown and cooked through, about 5-7 minutes per side. Season with salt and pepper to taste.

3. While the chicken is cooking, assemble the Greek yogurt bowls. Divide the remaining Greek yogurt among serving bowls.

4. Top the Greek yogurt with cooked chicken strips, halved cherry tomatoes, sliced red onion, and sliced bell peppers.

5. Drizzle the tzatziki sauce over the chicken and vegetables.

6. Garnish with additional chopped fresh dill and a squeeze of lemon juice if desired.

7. Serve immediately and enjoy your Greek yogurt bowls!

Nutritional Information (approx. per serving):

Calories: Around 350-400 calories

Protein: Approximately 35-40 grams

Fat: Approximately 10-15 grams

Carbohydrates: Around 20-25 grams

Fiber: Approximately 3-5 grams

SALMON BURGERS WITH AVOCADO CREMA AND WHOLE-WHEAT BUNS:

Prep Time: 15 minutes: Cooking Time: 10 minutes: Serving Size: 1 burger

Ingredients:

- 1 lb fresh salmon fillet, skin removed and chopped into small pieces
- 1/4 cup breadcrumbs (whole-wheat if available)
- 1/4 cup finely chopped red onion
- 2 tablespoons chopped fresh parsley
- 1 tablespoon lemon juice
- 1 teaspoon Dijon mustard

- 1 clove garlic, minced
- Salt and pepper to taste
- 4 whole-wheat burger buns
- 1 avocado, peeled and pitted
- 1/4 cup Greek yogurt (plain, unsweetened)
- 1 tablespoon lime juice
- 1 tablespoon chopped fresh cilantro
- Salt and pepper to taste
- Lettuce leaves, tomato slices, and additional toppings (optional)

Method of Preparation:

1. Preheat the grill or a grill pan over medium-high heat.
2. In a large mixing bowl, combine chopped salmon, breadcrumbs, chopped red onion, chopped parsley, lemon juice, Dijon mustard, minced garlic, salt, and pepper. Mix well until evenly combined.
3. Divide the salmon mixture into 4 equal portions and shape each portion into a burger patty.
4. Place the salmon burgers on the preheated grill or grill pan. Cook for about 4-5 minutes on each side, or until cooked through and nicely charred.
5. While the burgers are cooking, prepare the avocado crema. In a food processor or blender, combine peeled

and pitted avocado, Greek yogurt, lime juice, chopped cilantro, salt, and pepper. Blend until smooth and creamy.

6. Toast the whole-wheat burger buns on the grill for a minute or two until lightly toasted.
7. To assemble the burgers, spread a generous amount of avocado crema on the bottom half of each bun.
8. Place a cooked salmon burger on top of the avocado crema.
9. Add lettuce leaves, tomato slices, and any additional toppings of your choice.
10. Cover with the top half of the bun.
11. Serve immediately and enjoy your salmon burgers!

Nutritional Information (approx. per serving):

Calories: Around 350-400 calories (excluding additional toppings)

Protein: Approximately 25-30 grams

Fat: Approximately 15-20 grams

Carbohydrates: Around 30-35 grams

Fiber: Approximately 5-8 grams

Prep Time: 15 minutes: Cooking Time: 30 minutes: Serving Size: 1 cup

Ingredients:

- 1 lb ground turkey
- 1 onion, diced
- 2 cloves garlic, minced
- 1 bell pepper, diced
- 1 can (15 oz) kidney beans, drained and rinsed
- 1 can (14.5 oz) diced tomatoes
- 1 cup frozen corn kernels
- 2 cups chicken or vegetable broth
- 2 tablespoons tomato paste
- 1 tablespoon chili powder
- 1 teaspoon ground cumin
- 1/2 teaspoon smoked paprika
- Salt and pepper to taste
- Olive oil for cooking
- Optional toppings: shredded cheese, chopped green onions, sour cream, cilantro, avocado slices, lime wedges

Method of Preparation:

1. Heat a drizzle of olive oil in a large pot over medium heat. Add diced onion, minced garlic, and diced bell pepper. Cook until softened, about 5-7 minutes.

2. Add ground turkey to the pot, breaking it apart with a spoon. Cook until browned and cooked through.

3. Stir in chili powder, ground cumin, smoked paprika, salt, and pepper. Cook for another minute until fragrant.

4. Add diced tomatoes, drained kidney beans, frozen corn kernels, chicken or vegetable broth, and tomato paste to the pot. Stir to combine.

5. Bring the chili to a simmer, then reduce the heat to low. Let it simmer uncovered for about 20-25 minutes, stirring occasionally, until the flavors are well combined and the chili has thickened.

6. Taste and adjust seasoning as needed.

7. Serve hot, garnished with your choice of toppings such as shredded cheese, chopped green onions, sour cream, cilantro, avocado slices, or a squeeze of lime juice.

8. Enjoy your delicious turkey chili with kidney beans and corn!

Nutritional Information (approx. per serving):

Calories: Around 250-300 calories

Protein: Approximately 20-25 grams

Fat: Approximately 10-15 grams

Carbohydrates: Around 20-25 grams

Fiber: Approximately 5-8 grams

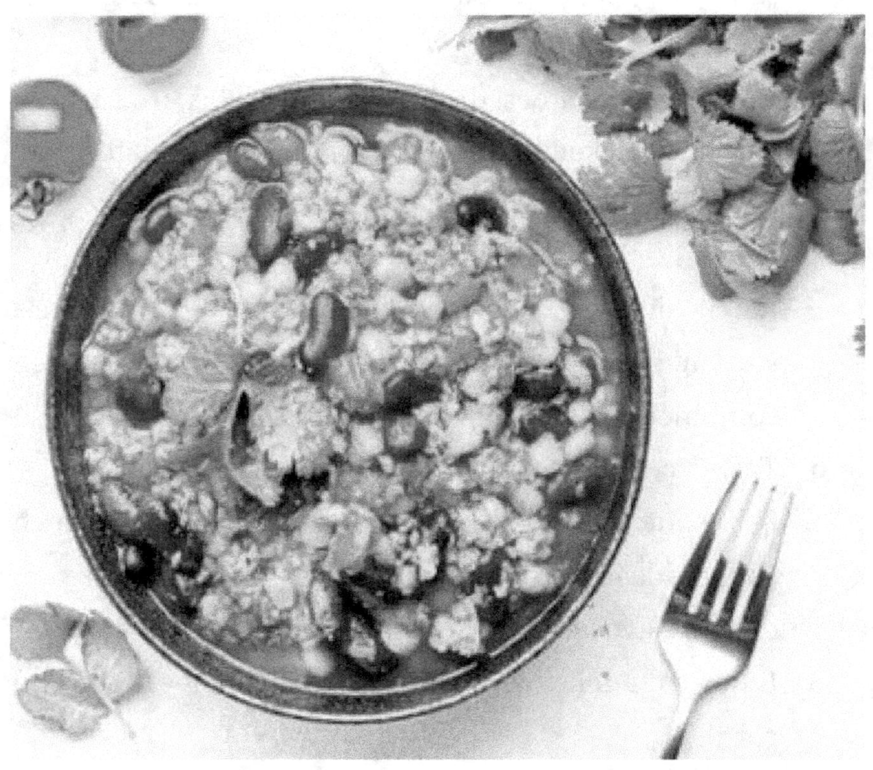

CHAPTER 9:

DESSERT RECIPES

Dark Chocolate with Berries and Nuts:

Ingredients:

- Dark chocolate (70% cocoa or higher)
- Assorted berries (such as strawberries, blueberries, raspberries)
- Assorted nuts (such as almonds, walnuts, pistachios)

Method of Preparation:

1. Melt dark chocolate in a microwave or using a double boiler until smooth.
2. Dip or drizzle berries and nuts with the melted dark chocolate.
3. Place them on a parchment-lined baking sheet and let them cool until the chocolate hardens.
4. Enjoy as a delicious and satisfying snack or dessert!

GREEK YOGURT WITH BERRIES AND CHIA SEEDS:

Ingredients:

- Greek yogurt (plain, unsweetened)
- Assorted berries (such as strawberries, blueberries, raspberries)
- Chia seeds

Method of Preparation:

1. Spoon Greek yogurt into a bowl or serving glass.
2. Top with fresh berries and sprinkle with chia seeds.
3. Enjoy this nutritious and protein-packed snack or breakfast option!

FROZEN BERRIES WITH COCONUT MILK:

Ingredients:

- Assorted frozen berries (such as strawberries, blueberries, blackberries)
- Coconut milk (canned or homemade)

Method of Preparation:

1. Place frozen berries in a bowl.

2. Pour coconut milk over the berries until they are coated.

3. Let them sit at room temperature for a few minutes until the coconut milk starts to slightly thaw and create a creamy texture.

4. Enjoy this refreshing and creamy treat as a healthy dessert or snack option!

BAKED APPLE WITH CINNAMON:

Ingredients:

- Apples (any variety)
- Ground cinnamon

Method of Preparation:

1. Preheat the oven to 375°F (190°C).

2. Core the apples and slice them horizontally into rings or cut them in half.

3. Place the apple slices on a baking sheet lined with parchment paper.

4. Sprinkle ground cinnamon over the apple slices.

5. Bake in the preheated oven for about 15-20 minutes, or until the apples are tender.

6. Serve warm as a healthy and delicious dessert or snack option!

HOMEMADE ENERGY BITES:

Ingredients:

- Rolled oats
- Nut butter (such as peanut butter, almond butter)
- Honey or maple syrup
- Optional mix-ins (such as chocolate chips, dried fruit, nuts, seeds)

Method of Preparation:

1. In a mixing bowl, combine rolled oats, nut butter, and honey or maple syrup.
2. Add optional mix-ins like chocolate chips, dried fruit, nuts, or seeds, if desired.
3. Mix until well combined and the mixture holds together.
4. Roll the mixture into small bite-sized balls using your hands.
5. Place the energy bites on a baking sheet lined with parchment paper.
6. Refrigerate for at least 30 minutes to firm up.
7. Enjoy these homemade energy bites as a convenient and nutritious snack on the go!

COTTAGE CHEESE WITH SLICED PEACHES:

Ingredients:

- Cottage cheese
- Ripe peaches, sliced

Method of Preparation:

1. Spoon cottage cheese into a bowl or serving dish.
2. Top with sliced ripe peaches.
3. Serve chilled or at room temperature as a refreshing and protein-packed snack or breakfast option!

SLICED CUCUMBER WITH MINT AND LIME:

Ingredients:
- Cucumber, sliced
- Fresh mint leaves, chopped
- Lime, sliced into wedges

Method of Preparation:
1. Arrange cucumber slices on a plate.
2. Sprinkle chopped fresh mint leaves over the cucumber slices.
3. Squeeze lime wedges over the cucumber slices.
4. Serve immediately as a light and refreshing snack or side dish!

AVOCADO CHOCOLATE MOUSSE:

Ingredients:

- 1 ripe avocado
- 2 tablespoons unsweetened cocoa powder
- 2 tablespoons maple syrup or honey
- 1/2 teaspoon vanilla extract
- Pinch of salt

Method of Preparation:

1. Scoop out the flesh of the avocado and place it in a blender or food processor.
2. Add cocoa powder, maple syrup or honey, vanilla extract, and a pinch of salt to the blender.
3. Blend until smooth and creamy, scraping down the sides of the blender as needed.
4. Transfer the avocado chocolate mousse to small serving dishes or ramekins.
5. Chill in the refrigerator for at least 30 minutes before serving.
6. Enjoy this indulgent and healthy dessert in limited quantities!

ROASTED PEARS WITH SPICES:

Ingredients:

- Pears (firm, ripe)
- Ground cinnamon
- Ground nutmeg
- Ground cloves
- Honey or maple syrup (optional)

Method of Preparation:

1. Preheat the oven to 375°F (190°C).
2. Cut the pears in half and remove the cores.
3. Place the pear halves cut-side up on a baking sheet lined with parchment paper.
4. Sprinkle ground cinnamon, ground nutmeg, and ground cloves over the pear halves.
5. Drizzle with honey or maple syrup if desired.
6. Roast in the preheated oven for 20-25 minutes, or until the pears are tender and caramelized.
7. Serve warm as a delicious dessert or snack option!

HOMEMADE YOGURT POPSICLES:

Ingredients:

- Greek yogurt (plain, unsweetened)
- Fresh fruit (such as berries, sliced bananas, diced mango)
- Honey or maple syrup (optional)

Method of Preparation:

1. In a bowl, mix Greek yogurt with honey or maple syrup if desired.
2. Spoon the yogurt mixture into popsicle molds, filling them halfway.
3. Add fresh fruit pieces to the molds, pressing them down gently into the yogurt.
4. Fill the molds with the remaining yogurt mixture, leaving a little space at the top.
5. Insert popsicle sticks into the molds.
6. Freeze for at least 4 hours, or until the yogurt popsicles are completely frozen.
7. To remove the popsicles from the molds, run them under warm water for a few seconds.
8. Enjoy these refreshing and nutritious homemade yogurt popsicles as a guilt-free treat!

CHAPTER 10:

JUICING FOR WEIGHT LOSS

GREEN GLOW:

Ingredients:

- Handful of spinach leaves
- 1/2 cucumber, chopped
- 1 celery stalk, chopped
- 1 apple (optional for sweetness), cored and chopped

Method of Preparation:

1. Place all ingredients in a blender.
2. Blend until smooth.
3. Adjust sweetness by adding more apple if desired.
4. Pour into a glass and enjoy!

TROPICAL GREEN:

Ingredients:

- Handful of kale leaves
- 1 cup pineapple chunks
- 1 teaspoon grated ginger

Method of Preparation:

1. Place all ingredients in a blender.
2. Blend until smooth.
3. Adjust consistency with water if needed.
4. Pour into a glass and enjoy the tropical flavors!

BEET BLAST:

Ingredients:

- 1 small beet, peeled and chopped
- 1 carrot, chopped
- 1 apple (optional for sweetness), cored and chopped

Method of Preparation:

1. Place all ingredients in a blender.
2. Blend until smooth.
3. Adjust sweetness by adding more apple if desired.
4. Pour into a glass and enjoy the vibrant color and flavors!

SPICY CARROT:

Ingredients:

- 2 carrots, chopped
- 1 teaspoon grated ginger
- Juice of 1 lemon

Method of Preparation:

1. Place all ingredients in a blender.
2. Blend until smooth.
3. Adjust consistency with water if needed.
4. Pour into a glass and enjoy the zesty kick!

ZUCCHINI ZING:

Ingredients:

- 1 small zucchini, chopped
- 1/2 cucumber, chopped
- Handful of fresh mint leaves

Method of Preparation:

1. Place all ingredients in a blender.
2. Blend until smooth.
3. Adjust consistency with water if needed.
4. Pour into a glass and enjoy the refreshing zing!

BERRY BLAST:

Ingredients:

- Mixed berries (such as strawberries, blueberries, raspberries, blackberries)

Method of Preparation:

1. Place the mixed berries in a blender.
2. Blend until smooth.
3. Optionally, add a splash of water or juice for desired consistency.
4. Pour into a glass and enjoy the burst of berry flavors!

CITRUS SUNRISE:

Ingredients:

- 1 orange, peeled and segmented
- 1/2 grapefruit, peeled and segmented
- 1 teaspoon grated ginger

Method of Preparation:

1. Place the orange segments, grapefruit segments, and grated ginger in a blender.
2. Blend until smooth.
3. Optionally, add a few ice cubes for a chilled smoothie.
4. Pour into a glass and savor the refreshing citrusy taste!

MELON MEDLEY:

Ingredients:

- Watermelon, cubed
- Cantaloupe, cubed
- Juice of 1 lime

Method of Preparation:

1. Place the cubed watermelon and cantaloupe in a blender.
2. Squeeze the lime juice over the melon.
3. Blend until smooth.
4. Optionally, add a sprig of mint for extra freshness.
5. Pour into a glass and enjoy the sweet and tangy melon flavors!

GREEN VEGGIE & APPLE:

Ingredients:

Assorted green vegetables (such as spinach, kale, cucumber)
1 small apple, cored and chopped
Method of Preparation:

1. Combine the green vegetables and chopped apple in a blender.
2. Blend until smooth.
3. Adjust sweetness by adding more apple if desired.
4. Optionally, add a squeeze of lemon juice for extra zing.
5. Pour into a glass and relish the green goodness!

VEGGIE & CITRUS:

Ingredients:

- Assorted vegetables (such as carrots, celery, cucumber)
- Juice of lemon or orange

Method of Preparation:

1. Mix the assorted vegetables with the juice of lemon or orange in a blender.
2. Blend until smooth.
3. Optionally, add a splash of water for desired consistency.
4. Pour into a glass and enjoy the vibrant and refreshing flavor!

TROPICAL PARADISE:

Ingredients:

- Pineapple chunks
- Mango chunks
- Handful of spinach leaves

Method of Preparation:

1. Place the pineapple chunks, mango chunks, and spinach leaves in a blender.
2. Blend until smooth.
3. Optionally, add coconut water or coconut milk for a tropical twist.
4. Pour into a glass and transport yourself to a tropical paradise with every sip!

CONCLUSION

In the journey of women over 40, intermittent fasting has been a game-changer—a simple yet powerful tool for reclaiming health and vitality. As we come to the end of this story, it's clear that intermittent fasting isn't just about losing weight or fitting into smaller clothes. It's about rediscovering our strength, resilience, and confidence.

Through intermittent fasting, women have found a new sense of control over their bodies and their lives. They've learned that hunger isn't something to fear but a signal of their body's amazing ability to adapt and thrive. With each fasting cycle, they've shed not only pounds but also self-doubt, embracing their bodies with gratitude and appreciation.

This journey isn't just about what happens on the outside. It's about the transformation that occurs within—a shift in mindset that empowers women to take charge of their health and well-being. It's about realizing that age is just a number and that it's never too late to make positive changes.

So, as we close this chapter, let's carry forward the lessons learned from intermittent fasting—a reminder that simple changes can lead to profound results.

Let's embrace our strength, celebrate our victories, and continue to write our own stories of health, happiness, and empowerment.

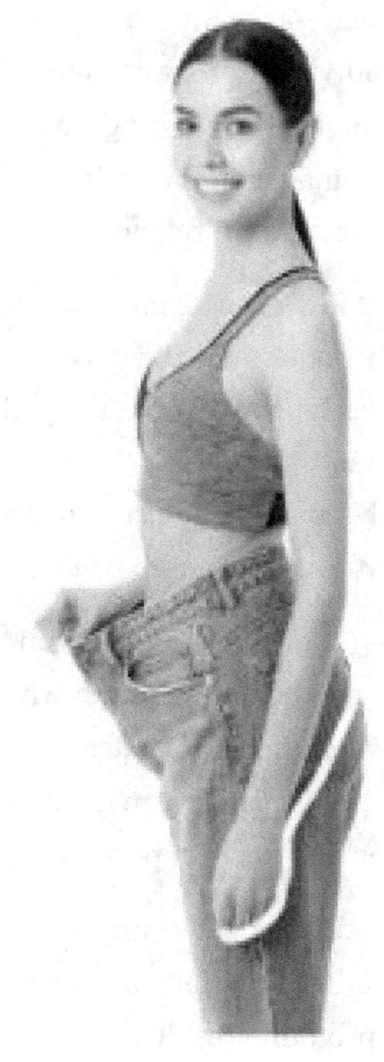